T0380697

A
New
Day
and a
New
Normal

A New Day and a New Normal

A Personal Journal for Breast Cancer Survivors

ROSEMARY R. KING APRN, BC

iUniverse

A NEW DAY AND A NEW NORMAL
A PERSONAL JOURNAL FOR BREAST CANCER SURVIVORS

iUniverse books may be ordered through booksellers or by contacting:

iUniverse
1663 Liberty Drive
Bloomington, IN 47403
www.iuniverse.com
1-800-Authors (1-800-288-4677)

ISBN: 978-1-5320-6075-5 (sc)
ISBN: 978-1-5320-6074-8 (e)

Library of Congress Control Number: 2018912594

Print information available on the last page.

iUniverse rev. date: 10/27/2018

To all the brave women who are battling this terrible disease
and to their families who are struggling alongside them

CONTENTS

CONTENTS

INTRODUCTION

My dear friend:

I am so sorry that you are now a part of this sisterhood. Not one of us thought that this would ever happen to us. Unfortunately, one in every eight women now is expected to be diagnosed with breast cancer.

As a nurse practitioner for the past forty years, I am a little more knowledgeable about cancer, but oncology has not been my specialty for many years. It quickly became apparent that many things have changed over the years, and it was imperative that I research as much as possible in order to take charge of my health and make responsible decisions and choices.

Changes in my appearance, energy level, family relations, and friendships have occurred that I was not prepared for. Surgical procedures on my breast brought about body image and sexual concerns. It is frightening, scary, and terrifying, all at the same time. There have been good days and some very bad days.

I have found it very helpful to keep a journal to document and detail my journey. You may have kept a diary when you were younger; this is no different. The release of your emotions in the written word can help you heal.

I am hopeful that keeping this journal will aid you in a healing journey by concentrating on both your physical and emotional health.

My thoughts and prayers are with you always.

Rosemary King, APRN, BC

WHY BOTHER TO JOURNAL?

What is journaling? *Journaling*, according to Susan Borkin, author of *The Healing Power of Writing: A Therapist's Guide to Using Journaling with Clients*, is "any type of writing or related expressive process used for the purposes of psychological healing or growth."

Remember when you were a young girl? You may have had a diary. Your "dear diary" captured events and emotions in your life. Now, with this devastating diagnosis, journaling your experience can actually be liberating. How do you feel? What are you going through with treatments, either chemotherapy and/or radiation? How have your relationships changed with the onset of your diagnosis? Who are your friends, I mean, real friends? How has your perspective on life changed? What is now important to you? What are you grateful for?

If you purchased this book, you have already chosen to journal. Now, decide how you want to use this book. It can be any way you want. There are *no* rules. Just let it flow. If you feel that drawing, rather than writing, will express how you feel on any given day, feel free to supplement your journal pages with a sketch. Any medium that helps you express yourself best is acceptable. The idea is to express your emotions. As you journal your way through this experience, you will notice yourself transitioning through the stages, especially when you reread your entries at a later date.

I would also advise you not to worry about the quality of your writing unless you plan to share it with others. This journal is for you and you alone.

I would also encourage you to write about the full range of your emotions, and not just negative. The more positive your thoughts, the better you will feel overall. It is well known that our thoughts can control our actions.

What kind of outcomes might you encounter by journaling? Women who expressed their emotions actually found that they reported fewer symptoms during their journey and saw their medical doctors less for cancer-related issues. They felt better physically and had a greater sense of overall health. Stress was lower. Perspectives on various issues were identified and sometimes altered as priorities were focused on and readdressed. Health trends were identified, including improved health over time. And another strong result was that women began to be grateful for what they had and the positive things in their lives.

Many women with this diagnosis begin anew, concentrating on taking the time for themselves and being more health conscious with their diet and exercise regimens. I have included health monitors in the daily journal, should you choose to incorporate them. I have found them to be very motivating to keep making changes to meet my goals.

I have also included several appendixes to include questions to ask your specialists, book references, websites, current Facebook support groups, apps for your phone, and a glossary of terms that you may encounter in your medical documentation. You are not alone, and there will be help and support along the way.

I wish you all the best in this journey.

WORKS CITED

Borkin, Susan. *The Healing Power of Writing: A Therapist's Guide to Using Journaling with Clients*. New York: Norton, 2014.

CANCER AND THE FIVE
STAGES OF GRIEF

I felt that it was helpful to address some of the roller coaster emotions that happen with cancer. Know that you are not alone. I dare say that all of us are touched by unexpected loss at some time in our lives. The diagnosis of cancer begins a whirlwind of emotions and the medical cavalcade of specialists, surgeries, treatments, and medications. The world that you have known is now different and will never be the same. You are experiencing a profound loss in your way of life and in your physical being. Reactions to these changes can be loosely predicted and are completely normal. It is also comforting to know that millions of people have experienced this and have come to a personal acceptance of the loss. As you journal your way through this experience, you will notice the transitioning through the stages, especially when you reread your entries at a later date.

You may recall, from years ago, the esteemed Swiss-born doctor Dr. Elisabeth Kübler-Ross, who identified the five stages of grief in her famous book, *On Death and Dying*. It was initially relating to the awareness of one's own impending death, but these concepts have broadened to cover all those suffering from a significant loss of something very important to them. It is important to note that not everyone goes through all five stages. Some even go back and forth through the stages in a different order. Grieving is a very individual process. So what are the stages of grief?

1. **Denial:** This, by far, is usually the first reaction. "This can't be happening to me; no, they are wrong." It may be more difficult to accept if the incident was totally unexpected or sudden. It is not uncommon for people to go from one doctor to another just hoping that the diagnosis was wrong. This feeling of shock and numbness is your body's defense mechanism toward this overwhelming emotion. Individuals may withdraw from their normal habits and avoid social interaction. Denial has no set time frame.

2. **Anger, blame, or guilt:** Once the reality that this is happening becomes clear, it is normal to become angry, even very angry. It is also common to look for blame and then to feel self-guilt. Whose fault is it? "Why did this happen to me?" If only, if only, if only. It is not uncommon to direct your anger at those that you love, or at God, if you so believe. Just realize that this is a normal process.

3. **Bargaining:** Some people may find themselves bargaining: bargaining with God, bargaining with their spouses, promising to do better from now on—eating better, stopping smoking, stopping gambling, or stopping whatever they feel may have contributed to the issue at hand. It is actually a positive stage because you are moving toward the reality of the situation. Once the true reality sets in, the next stage may be depression.

4. **Depression:** This is when things really hit you and the reality of your situation becomes crystal clear. This is a time when you may cry, shout, withdraw from others, lash out, and feel totally helpless and hopeless. Sleep disturbances, as well as changes in eating patterns, may arise. Feelings of being overwhelmed are common, and suicidal thoughts may surface as a sense of finality sets in. Professional help may be invaluable to those who are struggling with this stage.

5. **Acceptance:** This is the final stage, when you accept the loss of your past life and are ready to move on to a new point in your life, a new beginning. This is not to say that things will be normal again, but they will settle into a new normal.

Here are a few ideas to help you cope with these stages:

- There is no specific time limit for the grieving process. Give yourself time and permission to grieve.
- Do not isolate yourself from friends and family. Now is the time to seek support from those who care about you.
- Learn everything you can about your particular diagnosis and options so that you are in control of the final decision-making process and feel good about those decisions.
- Partner with good medical providers who are willing to listen to you and provide answers to your questions. Do not be afraid to seek second or third opinions before making treatment choices.

ROSEMARY R. KING APRN, BC

- Continue doing what is important to you and any activities or hobbies that give you joy.
- Concentrate on healthful activities, such as whole food nutrition, exercising, decreasing stress, and sound sleep.
- Choose support groups that mirror your particular situation.

There will be times when new issues arise and the feelings will bounce back and forth among the stages. This may occur with an anniversary date or when a particular song plays on the radio. It is normal, natural, and healthy. Do not get discouraged.

MY PERSONAL INFORMATION

Name:_____

Diagnosis:_____

Date of diagnosis:_____

Cancer type/location/histology:_____

Stage: 0_____1_____2_____3_____4_____ NA_____

Surgery: Yes_____ No_____ Date(s):_____

Surgical procedure:_____

Radiation: Yes_____ No_____ Body area treated:_____

Systemic Therapy (chemotherapy, hormonal therapy, other): Yes No

Agents used:_____

_____

_____

Record of Diagnostic Testing

Type   Date   Outcome

_____

_____

_____

Genetic/hereditary testing:_____

ROSEMARY R. KING APRN, BC

IMPORTANT CONTACTS

Primary support person:_____ Relationship:_____

Phone (cell/home/work):_____

Primary care provider:_____

Phone/email:_____

Primary oncologist:_____

Phone/email:_____

Radiation oncologist:_____

Phone/email:_____

Surgeon:_____

Phone/email:_____

GYN provider:_____

Phone/email:_____

Other providers, such as naturopath or
functional medicine:_____

Phone/email:_____

MY JOURNEY

Date:_____Weight:_____BP:_____

Blood sugar level:_____ Hours slept last night:_____

If using a FitBit or other device, number of steps taken today: _____

Exercise: Aerobic_____ Strengthening_____

In general, today I feel: Good_____ Fair_____ Poor_____

Pain level (0–10):_____

Drugs/Medications:_____
_____
_____
_____

Vitamins/Herbs:_____
_____
_____
_____

Today's Diet

Breakfast:_____
_____
_____
_____
_____

Lunch:_____
_____
_____
_____

Dinner:_____
_____
_____
_____

Snacks:_____

_____

Thoughts and Feelings Today

_____
_____
_____
_____
_____
_____
_____
_____
_____
_____
_____
_____
_____
_____
_____
_____
_____
_____
_____
_____
_____
_____
_____
_____
_____
_____

ROSEMARY R. KING APRN, BC

Date:_____Weight:_____BP:_____

Blood sugar level:_____ Hours slept last night:_____

If using a FitBit or other device, number of steps taken today: _____

Exercise: Aerobic_____ Strengthening_____

In general, today I feel: Good_____ Fair_____ Poor_____

Pain level (0–10):_____

Drugs/Medications:_____

_____

_____

_____

Vitamins/Herbs:_____

_____

_____

_____

Today's Diet

Breakfast:_____

_____

_____

_____

_____

Lunch:_____

_____

_____

_____

Dinner:_____

_____

_____

_____

Snacks:_____

_____

_____

Thoughts and Feelings Today

_____

_____

_____

_____

_____

_____

_____

_____

_____

_____

_____

_____

_____

_____

_____

_____

_____

_____

_____

_____

_____

_____

_____

_____

ROSEMARY R. KING APRN, BC

Date:_____Weight:_____BP:_____

Blood sugar level:_____ Hours slept last night:_____

If using a FitBit or other device, number of steps taken today: _____

Exercise: Aerobic_____ Strengthening_____

In general, today I feel: Good_____ Fair_____ Poor_____

Pain level (0–10):_____

Drugs/Medications:_____

_____

_____

_____

Vitamins/Herbs:_____

_____

_____

_____

Today's Diet

Breakfast:_____

_____

_____

_____

_____

Lunch:_____

_____

_____

_____

Dinner:_____

_____

_____

_____

Snacks:_____
_____
_____

Thoughts and Feelings Today

_____
_____
_____
_____
_____
_____
_____
_____
_____
_____
_____
_____
_____
_____
_____
_____
_____
_____
_____
_____
_____
_____
_____
_____
_____
_____

ROSEMARY R. KING APRN, BC

Date:_____Weight:_____BP:_____

Blood sugar level:_____ Hours slept last night:_____

If using a FitBit or other device, number of steps taken today: _____

Exercise: Aerobic_____ Strengthening_____

In general, today I feel: Good_____ Fair_____ Poor_____

Pain level (0–10):_____

Drugs/Medications:_____
_____
_____
_____

Vitamins/Herbs:_____
_____
_____
_____

Today's Diet

Breakfast:_____
_____
_____
_____

Lunch:_____
_____
_____
_____

Dinner:_____
_____
_____
_____

Snacks:_____

_____

_____

Thoughts and Feelings Today

_____

_____

_____

_____

_____

_____

_____

_____

_____

_____

_____

_____

_____

_____

_____

_____

_____

_____

_____

_____

_____

_____

_____

_____

_____

_____

_____

ROSEMARY R. KING APRN, BC

Date:_____ Weight:_____ BP:_____

Blood sugar level:_____ Hours slept last night:_____

If using a FitBit or other device, number of steps taken today: _____

Exercise: Aerobic_____ Strengthening_____

In general, today I feel: Good_____ Fair_____ Poor_____

Pain level (0–10):_____

Drugs/Medications:_____

_____

_____

_____

Vitamins/Herbs:_____

_____

_____

_____

Today's Diet

Breakfast:_____

_____

_____

_____

_____

Lunch:_____

_____

_____

_____

Dinner:_____

_____

_____

_____

Snacks:_____
_____

Thoughts and Feelings Today

_____
_____
_____
_____
_____
_____
_____
_____
_____
_____
_____
_____
_____
_____
_____
_____
_____
_____
_____
_____
_____
_____
_____
_____
_____
_____
_____

ROSEMARY R. KING APRN, BC

Date:_____Weight:_____BP:_____

Blood sugar level:_____ Hours slept last night:_____

If using a FitBit or other device, number of steps taken today: _____

Exercise: Aerobic_____ Strengthening_____

In general, today I feel: Good_____ Fair_____ Poor_____

Pain level (0–10):_____

Drugs/Medications:_____
_____
_____
_____

Vitamins/Herbs:_____
_____
_____
_____

Today's Diet

Breakfast:_____
_____
_____
_____
_____

Lunch:_____
_____
_____
_____

Dinner:_____
_____
_____
_____

Snacks:_____

_____

Thoughts and Feelings Today

_____
_____
_____
_____
_____
_____
_____
_____
_____
_____
_____
_____
_____
_____
_____
_____
_____
_____
_____
_____
_____
_____
_____
_____
_____

Date:_____Weight:_____BP:_____

Blood sugar level:_____ Hours slept last night:_____

If using a FitBit or other device, number of steps taken today: _____

Exercise: Aerobic_____ Strengthening_____

In general, today I feel: Good_____ Fair_____ Poor_____

Pain level (0–10):_____

Drugs/Medications:_____

_____

_____

_____

Vitamins/Herbs:_____

_____

_____

_____

Today's Diet

Breakfast:_____

_____

_____

_____

Lunch:_____

_____

_____

_____

Dinner:_____

_____

_____

_____

Snacks:_____

_____

Thoughts and Feelings Today

_____

_____

_____

_____

_____

_____

_____

_____

_____

_____

_____

_____

_____

_____

_____

_____

_____

_____

_____

_____

_____

_____

ROSEMARY R. KING APRN, BC

Date:_____Weight:_____BP:_____

Blood sugar level:_____ Hours slept last night:_____

If using a FitBit or other device, number of steps taken today: _____

Exercise: Aerobic_____ Strengthening_____

In general, today I feel: Good_____ Fair_____ Poor_____

Pain level (0–10):_____

Drugs/Medications:_____
_____
_____
_____

Vitamins/Herbs:_____
_____
_____
_____

Today's Diet

Breakfast:_____
_____
_____
_____
_____

Lunch:_____
_____
_____
_____

Dinner:_____
_____
_____
_____

Snacks:_____
_____
_____

Thoughts and Feelings Today

_____
_____
_____
_____
_____
_____
_____
_____
_____
_____
_____
_____
_____
_____
_____
_____
_____
_____
_____
_____
_____
_____
_____
_____
_____
_____

ROSEMARY R. KING APRN, BC

Date:_____Weight:_____BP:_____

Blood sugar level:_____ Hours slept last night:_____

If using a FitBit or other device, number of steps taken today: _____

Exercise: Aerobic_____ Strengthening_____

In general, today I feel: Good_____ Fair_____ Poor_____

Pain level (0–10):_____

Drugs/Medications:_____
_____
_____
_____

Vitamins/Herbs:_____
_____
_____
_____

Today's Diet

Breakfast:_____
_____
_____
_____
_____

Lunch:_____
_____
_____
_____

Dinner:_____
_____
_____
_____

Snacks:_____

_____

_____

Thoughts and Feelings Today

_____

_____

_____

_____

_____

_____

_____

_____

_____

_____

_____

_____

_____

_____

_____

_____

_____

_____

_____

_____

_____

_____

_____

_____

_____

ROSEMARY R. KING APRN, BC

Date:_____ Weight:_____ BP:_____

Blood sugar level:_____ Hours slept last night:_____

If using a FitBit or other device, number of steps taken today: _____

Exercise: Aerobic_____ Strengthening_____

In general, today I feel: Good_____ Fair_____ Poor_____

Pain level (0–10):_____

Drugs/Medications:_____

_____

_____

_____

Vitamins/Herbs:_____

_____

_____

_____

Today's Diet

Breakfast:_____

_____

_____

_____

_____

Lunch:_____

_____

_____

_____

Dinner:_____

_____

_____

_____

Snacks:_____

_____

Thoughts and Feelings Today

_____

_____

_____

_____

_____

_____

_____

_____

_____

_____

_____

_____

_____

_____

_____

_____

_____

_____

_____

_____

_____

_____

_____

_____

_____

ROSEMARY R. KING APRN, BC

Date:_____Weight:_____BP:_____

Blood sugar level:_____ Hours slept last night:_____

If using a FitBit or other device, number of steps taken today: _____

Exercise: Aerobic_____ Strengthening_____

In general, today I feel: Good_____ Fair_____ Poor_____

Pain level (0–10):_____

Drugs/Medications:_____
_____
_____
_____

Vitamins/Herbs:_____
_____
_____
_____

Today's Diet

Breakfast:_____
_____
_____
_____
_____

Lunch:_____
_____
_____
_____

Dinner:_____
_____
_____
_____

Snacks:_____

_____

Thoughts and Feelings Today

_____
_____
_____
_____
_____
_____
_____
_____
_____
_____
_____
_____
_____
_____
_____
_____
_____
_____
_____
_____
_____
_____
_____
_____
_____
_____
_____
_____

Date:_____Weight:_____BP:_____

Blood sugar level:_____ Hours slept last night:_____

If using a FitBit or other device, number of steps taken today: _____

Exercise: Aerobic_____ Strengthening_____

In general, today I feel: Good_____ Fair_____ Poor_____

Pain level (0–10):_____

Drugs/Medications:_____

_____

_____

_____

Vitamins/Herbs:_____

_____

_____

_____

Today's Diet

Breakfast:_____

_____

_____

_____

_____

Lunch:_____

_____

_____

_____

Dinner:_____

_____

_____

_____

Snacks:_____

_____

_____

Thoughts and Feelings Today

_____

_____

_____

_____

_____

_____

_____

_____

_____

_____

_____

_____

_____

_____

_____

_____

_____

_____

_____

_____

_____

_____

_____

_____

_____

_____

ROSEMARY R. KING APRN, BC

Date:_____Weight:_____BP:_____

Blood sugar level:_____ Hours slept last night:_____

If using a FitBit or other device, number of steps taken today: _____

Exercise: Aerobic_____ Strengthening_____

In general, today I feel: Good_____ Fair_____ Poor_____

Pain level (0–10):_____

Drugs/Medications:_____
_____
_____
_____

Vitamins/Herbs:_____
_____
_____
_____

Today's Diet

Breakfast:_____
_____
_____
_____
_____

Lunch:_____
_____
_____
_____

Dinner:_____
_____
_____
_____

Snacks:_____

_____

_____

Thoughts and Feelings Today

_____

_____

_____

_____

_____

_____

_____

_____

_____

_____

_____

_____

_____

_____

_____

_____

_____

_____

_____

_____

_____

_____

_____

_____

_____

_____

ROSEMARY R. KING APRN, BC

Date:_____Weight:_____BP:_____

Blood sugar level:_____ Hours slept last night:_____

If using a FitBit or other device, number of steps taken today: _____

Exercise: Aerobic_____ Strengthening_____

In general, today I feel: Good_____ Fair_____ Poor_____

Pain level (0–10):_____

Drugs/Medications:_____

_____

_____

_____

Vitamins/Herbs:_____

_____

_____

_____

Today's Diet

Breakfast:_____

_____

_____

_____

_____

Lunch:_____

_____

_____

_____

Dinner:_____

_____

_____

_____

Snacks:_____

_____

Thoughts and Feelings Today

_____
_____
_____
_____
_____
_____
_____
_____
_____
_____
_____
_____
_____
_____
_____
_____
_____
_____
_____
_____
_____
_____
_____
_____
_____
_____
_____

Date:_____Weight:_____BP:_____

Blood sugar level:_____ Hours slept last night:_____

If using a FitBit or other device, number of steps taken today: _____

Exercise: Aerobic_____ Strengthening_____

In general, today I feel: Good_____ Fair_____ Poor_____

Pain level (0–10):_____

Drugs/Medications:_____
_____
_____
_____

Vitamins/Herbs:_____
_____
_____
_____

Today's Diet

Breakfast:_____
_____
_____
_____

Lunch:_____
_____
_____
_____

Dinner:_____
_____
_____
_____

Snacks:_____

_____

_____

Thoughts and Feelings Today

_____

_____

_____

_____

_____

_____

_____

_____

_____

_____

_____

_____

_____

_____

_____

_____

_____

_____

_____

_____

_____

_____

_____

Date:_____Weight:_____BP:_____

Blood sugar level:_____ Hours slept last night:_____

If using a FitBit or other device, number of steps taken today: _____

Exercise: Aerobic_____ Strengthening_____

In general, today I feel: Good_____ Fair_____ Poor_____

Pain level (0–10):_____

Drugs/Medications:_____
_____
_____
_____

Vitamins/Herbs:_____
_____
_____
_____

Today's Diet

Breakfast:_____
_____
_____
_____

Lunch:_____
_____
_____
_____

Dinner:_____
_____
_____
_____

Snacks:_____

_____

_____

Thoughts and Feelings Today

_____

_____

_____

_____

_____

_____

_____

_____

_____

_____

_____

_____

_____

_____

_____

_____

_____

_____

_____

_____

_____

_____

_____

_____

_____

_____

Date:_____ Weight:_____ BP:_____

Blood sugar level:_____ Hours slept last night:_____

If using a FitBit or other device, number of steps taken today: _____

Exercise: Aerobic_____ Strengthening_____

In general, today I feel: Good_____ Fair_____ Poor_____

Pain level (0–10):_____

Drugs/Medications:_____
_____
_____
_____

Vitamins/Herbs:_____
_____
_____
_____

Today's Diet

Breakfast:_____
_____
_____
_____
_____

Lunch:_____
_____
_____
_____

Dinner:_____
_____
_____
_____

Snacks:_____

_____

_____

Thoughts and Feelings Today

_____

_____

_____

_____

_____

_____

_____

_____

_____

_____

_____

_____

_____

_____

_____

_____

_____

_____

_____

_____

_____

_____

_____

_____

_____

Date:_____ Weight:_____ BP:_____

Blood sugar level:_____ Hours slept last night:_____

If using a FitBit or other device, number of steps taken today: _____

Exercise: Aerobic_____ Strengthening_____

In general, today I feel: Good_____ Fair_____ Poor_____

Pain level (0–10):_____

Drugs/Medications:_____

_____

_____

_____

Vitamins/Herbs:_____

_____

_____

_____

Today's Diet

Breakfast:_____

_____

_____

_____

Lunch:_____

_____

_____

_____

Dinner:_____

_____

_____

_____

Snacks:_____

_____

Thoughts and Feelings Today

_____
_____
_____
_____
_____
_____
_____
_____
_____
_____
_____
_____
_____
_____
_____
_____
_____
_____
_____
_____
_____
_____
_____
_____
_____
_____

Date:_____Weight:_____BP:_____

Blood sugar level:_____ Hours slept last night:_____

If using a FitBit or other device, number of steps taken today: _____

Exercise: Aerobic_____ Strengthening_____

In general, today I feel: Good_____ Fair_____ Poor_____

Pain level (0–10):_____

Drugs/Medications:_____

_____

_____

_____

Vitamins/Herbs:_____

_____

_____

_____

Today's Diet

Breakfast:_____

_____

_____

_____

Lunch:_____

_____

_____

Dinner:_____

_____

_____

_____

Snacks:_____

_____

Thoughts and Feelings Today

_____
_____
_____
_____
_____
_____
_____
_____
_____
_____
_____
_____
_____
_____
_____
_____
_____
_____
_____
_____
_____
_____
_____
_____

ROSEMARY R. KING APRN, BC

Date:_____Weight:_____BP:_____

Blood sugar level:_____ Hours slept last night:_____

If using a FitBit or other device, number of steps taken today: _____

Exercise: Aerobic_____ Strengthening_____

In general, today I feel: Good_____ Fair_____ Poor_____

Pain level (0–10):_____

Drugs/Medications:_____

_____

_____

_____

Vitamins/Herbs:_____

_____

_____

_____

Today's Diet

Breakfast:_____

_____

_____

_____

_____

Lunch:_____

_____

_____

_____

Dinner:_____

_____

_____

_____

Snacks:_____

_____

Thoughts and Feelings Today

_____
_____
_____
_____
_____
_____
_____
_____
_____
_____
_____
_____
_____
_____
_____
_____
_____
_____
_____
_____
_____
_____
_____
_____
_____

ROSEMARY R. KING APRN, BC

Date:_____Weight:_____BP:_____

Blood sugar level:_____ Hours slept last night:_____

If using a FitBit or other device, number of steps taken today: _____

Exercise: Aerobic_____ Strengthening_____

In general, today I feel: Good_____ Fair_____ Poor_____

Pain level (0–10):_____

Drugs/Medications:_____
_____
_____
_____

Vitamins/Herbs:_____
_____
_____
_____

Today's Diet

Breakfast:_____
_____
_____
_____
_____

Lunch:_____
_____
_____
_____

Dinner:_____
_____
_____
_____

Snacks:_____

_____

_____

Thoughts and Feelings Today

_____

_____

_____

_____

_____

_____

_____

_____

_____

_____

_____

_____

_____

_____

_____

_____

_____

_____

_____

_____

_____

_____

_____

_____

ROSEMARY R. KING APRN, BC

Date:_____Weight:_____BP:_____

Blood sugar level:_____ Hours slept last night:_____

If using a FitBit or other device, number of steps taken today: _____

Exercise: Aerobic_____ Strengthening_____

In general, today I feel: Good_____ Fair_____ Poor_____

Pain level (0–10):_____

Drugs/Medications:_____
_____
_____
_____

Vitamins/Herbs:_____
_____
_____
_____

Today's Diet

Breakfast:_____
_____
_____
_____
_____

Lunch:_____
_____
_____
_____

Dinner:_____
_____
_____
_____

Snacks:_____

_____

Thoughts and Feelings Today

ROSEMARY R. KING APRN, BC

Date:_____ Weight:_____ BP:_____

Blood sugar level:_____ Hours slept last night:_____

If using a FitBit or other device, number of steps taken today: _____

Exercise: Aerobic_____ Strengthening_____

In general, today I feel: Good_____ Fair_____ Poor_____

Pain level (0–10):_____

Drugs/Medications:_____
_____
_____
_____

Vitamins/Herbs:_____
_____
_____
_____

Today's Diet

Breakfast:_____
_____
_____
_____
_____

Lunch:_____
_____
_____
_____

Dinner:_____
_____
_____
_____

Snacks:_____

_____

Thoughts and Feelings Today

_____
_____
_____
_____
_____
_____
_____
_____
_____
_____
_____
_____
_____
_____
_____
_____
_____
_____
_____
_____
_____
_____
_____
_____

ROSEMARY R. KING APRN, BC

Date:_____ Weight:_____ BP:_____

Blood sugar level:_____ Hours slept last night:_____

If using a FitBit or other device, number of steps taken today: _____

Exercise: Aerobic_____ Strengthening_____

In general, today I feel: Good_____ Fair_____ Poor_____

Pain level (0–10):_____

Drugs/Medications:_____
_____
_____
_____

Vitamins/Herbs:_____
_____
_____
_____

Today's Diet

Breakfast:_____
_____
_____
_____
_____

Lunch:_____
_____
_____
_____
_____

Dinner:_____
_____
_____
_____

Snacks:_____

_____

_____

Thoughts and Feelings Today

_____

_____

_____

_____

_____

_____

_____

_____

_____

_____

_____

_____

_____

_____

_____

_____

_____

_____

_____

_____

_____

_____

_____

_____

ROSEMARY R. KING APRN, BC

Date:_____Weight:_____BP:_____

Blood sugar level:_____ Hours slept last night:_____

If using a FitBit or other device, number of steps taken today: _____

Exercise: Aerobic_____ Strengthening_____

In general, today I feel: Good_____ Fair_____ Poor_____

Pain level (0–10):_____

Drugs/Medications:_____

_____

_____

_____

Vitamins/Herbs:_____

_____

_____

_____

Today's Diet

Breakfast:_____

_____

_____

_____

Lunch:_____

_____

_____

Dinner:_____

_____

_____

_____

Snacks:_____

_____

_____

Thoughts and Feelings Today

_____

_____

_____

_____

_____

_____

_____

_____

_____

_____

_____

_____

_____

_____

_____

_____

_____

_____

_____

_____

_____

_____

_____

_____

_____

_____

Date:_____Weight:_____BP:_____

Blood sugar level:_____ Hours slept last night:_____

If using a FitBit or other device, number of steps taken today: _____

Exercise: Aerobic_____ Strengthening_____

In general, today I feel: Good_____ Fair_____ Poor_____

Pain level (0–10):_____

Drugs/Medications:_____

_____

_____

_____

Vitamins/Herbs:_____

_____

_____

_____

Today's Diet

Breakfast:_____

_____

_____

_____

_____

Lunch:_____

_____

_____

_____

Dinner:_____

_____

_____

_____

Snacks:_____
_____
_____

Thoughts and Feelings Today

_____
_____
_____
_____
_____
_____
_____
_____
_____
_____
_____
_____
_____
_____
_____
_____
_____
_____
_____
_____
_____
_____
_____
_____
_____

ROSEMARY R. KING APRN, BC

Date:_____ Weight:_____ BP:_____

Blood sugar level:_____ Hours slept last night:_____

If using a FitBit or other device, number of steps taken today: _____

Exercise: Aerobic_____ Strengthening_____

In general, today I feel: Good_____ Fair_____ Poor_____

Pain level (0–10):_____

Drugs/Medications:_____

_____

_____

_____

Vitamins/Herbs:_____

_____

_____

_____

Today's Diet

Breakfast:_____

_____

_____

_____

_____

Lunch:_____

_____

_____

_____

Dinner:_____

_____

_____

_____

Snacks:_____

_____

Thoughts and Feelings Today

_____

_____

_____

_____

_____

_____

_____

_____

_____

_____

_____

_____

_____

_____

_____

_____

_____

_____

_____

_____

_____

_____

_____

_____

_____

_____

_____

_____

ROSEMARY R. KING APRN, BC

Date:_____Weight:_____BP:_____

Blood sugar level:_____ Hours slept last night:_____

If using a FitBit or other device, number of steps taken today: _____

Exercise: Aerobic_____ Strengthening_____

In general, today I feel: Good_____ Fair_____ Poor_____

Pain level (0–10):_____

Drugs/Medications:_____
_____
_____
_____

Vitamins/Herbs:_____
_____
_____
_____

Today's Diet

Breakfast:_____
_____
_____
_____
_____

Lunch:_____
_____
_____
_____

Dinner:_____
_____
_____
_____

Snacks:_____
_____
_____

Thoughts and Feelings Today

_____
_____
_____
_____
_____
_____
_____
_____
_____
_____
_____
_____
_____
_____
_____
_____
_____
_____
_____
_____
_____
_____
_____
_____
_____
_____

Date:_____Weight:_____BP:_____

Blood sugar level:_____ Hours slept last night:_____

If using a FitBit or other device, number of steps taken today: _____

Exercise: Aerobic_____ Strengthening_____

In general, today I feel: Good_____ Fair_____ Poor_____

Pain level (0–10):_____

Drugs/Medications:_____

_____

_____

_____

Vitamins/Herbs:_____

_____

_____

_____

Today's Diet

Breakfast:_____

_____

_____

_____

_____

Lunch:_____

_____

_____

_____

Dinner:_____

_____

_____

_____

Snacks:_____

_____

Thoughts and Feelings Today

_____

_____

_____

_____

_____

_____

_____

_____

_____

_____

_____

_____

_____

_____

_____

_____

_____

_____

_____

_____

_____

_____

_____

_____

_____

ROSEMARY R. KING APRN, BC

Date:_____Weight:_____BP:_____

Blood sugar level:_____ Hours slept last night:_____

If using a FitBit or other device, number of steps taken today: _____

Exercise: Aerobic_____ Strengthening_____

In general, today I feel: Good_____ Fair_____ Poor_____

Pain level (0–10):_____

Drugs/Medications:_____
_____
_____
_____

Vitamins/Herbs:_____
_____
_____
_____

Today's Diet

Breakfast:_____
_____
_____
_____
_____

Lunch:_____
_____
_____
_____

Dinner:_____
_____
_____
_____

Snacks:_____

_____

_____

Thoughts and Feelings Today

_____

_____

_____

_____

_____

_____

_____

_____

_____

_____

_____

_____

_____

_____

_____

_____

_____

_____

_____

_____

_____

_____

_____

ROSEMARY R. KING APRN, BC

Date:_____Weight:_____BP:_____

Blood sugar level:_____ Hours slept last night:_____

If using a FitBit or other device, number of steps taken today: _____

Exercise: Aerobic_____ Strengthening_____

In general, today I feel: Good_____ Fair_____ Poor_____

Pain level (0–10):_____

Drugs/Medications:_____

_____

_____

_____

Vitamins/Herbs:_____

_____

_____

_____

Today's Diet

Breakfast:_____

_____

_____

_____

_____

Lunch:_____

_____

_____

_____

Dinner:_____

_____

_____

_____

Snacks:_____

_____

_____

Thoughts and Feelings Today

_____

_____

_____

_____

_____

_____

_____

_____

_____

_____

_____

_____

_____

_____

_____

_____

_____

_____

_____

_____

_____

_____

_____

_____

_____

_____

_____

_____

ROSEMARY R. KING APRN, BC

Date:_____Weight:_____BP:_____

Blood sugar level:_____ Hours slept last night:_____

If using a FitBit or other device, number of steps taken today: _____

Exercise: Aerobic_____ Strengthening_____

In general, today I feel: Good_____ Fair_____ Poor_____

Pain level (0–10):_____

Drugs/Medications:_____

_____

_____

_____

Vitamins/Herbs:_____

_____

_____

_____

Today's Diet

Breakfast:_____

_____

_____

_____

_____

Lunch:_____

_____

_____

_____

Dinner:_____

_____

_____

_____

Snacks:_____

_____

Thoughts and Feelings Today

_____
_____
_____
_____
_____
_____
_____
_____
_____
_____
_____
_____
_____
_____
_____
_____
_____
_____
_____
_____
_____
_____
_____

ROSEMARY R. KING APRN, BC

Date:_____Weight:_____BP:_____

Blood sugar level:_____ Hours slept last night:_____

If using a FitBit or other device, number of steps taken today: _____

Exercise: Aerobic_____ Strengthening_____

In general, today I feel: Good_____ Fair_____ Poor_____

Pain level (0–10):_____

Drugs/Medications:_____
_____
_____
_____

Vitamins/Herbs:_____
_____
_____
_____

Today's Diet

Breakfast:_____
_____
_____
_____
_____

Lunch:_____
_____
_____
_____

Dinner:_____
_____
_____
_____

Snacks:_____

_____

_____

Thoughts and Feelings Today

_____

_____

_____

_____

_____

_____

_____

_____

_____

_____

_____

_____

_____

_____

_____

_____

_____

_____

_____

_____

_____

_____

_____

_____

_____

ROSEMARY R. KING APRN, BC

Date:_____Weight:_____BP:_____

Blood sugar level:_____ Hours slept last night:_____

If using a FitBit or other device, number of steps taken today: _____

Exercise: Aerobic_____ Strengthening_____

In general, today I feel: Good_____ Fair_____ Poor_____

Pain level (0–10):_____

Drugs/Medications:_____

_____

_____

_____

Vitamins/Herbs:_____

_____

_____

_____

Today's Diet

Breakfast:_____

_____

_____

_____

_____

Lunch:_____

_____

_____

_____

Dinner:_____

_____

_____

_____

Snacks:_____
_____

Thoughts and Feelings Today

_____
_____
_____
_____
_____
_____
_____
_____
_____
_____
_____
_____
_____
_____
_____
_____
_____
_____
_____
_____
_____
_____
_____

ROSEMARY R. KING APRN, BC

Date:_____ Weight:_____ BP:_____

Blood sugar level:_____ Hours slept last night:_____

If using a FitBit or other device, number of steps taken today: _____

Exercise: Aerobic_____ Strengthening_____

In general, today I feel: Good_____ Fair_____ Poor_____

Pain level (0–10):_____

Drugs/Medications:_____

_____

_____

_____

Vitamins/Herbs:_____

_____

_____

_____

Today's Diet

Breakfast:_____

_____

_____

_____

_____

Lunch:_____

_____

_____

_____

Dinner:_____

_____

_____

_____

Snacks:_____

_____

_____

Thoughts and Feelings Today

_____
_____
_____
_____
_____
_____
_____
_____
_____
_____
_____
_____
_____
_____
_____
_____
_____
_____
_____
_____
_____
_____
_____
_____
_____
_____
_____
_____
_____

Date:_____ Weight:_____ BP:_____

Blood sugar level:_____ Hours slept last night:_____

If using a FitBit or other device, number of steps taken today: _____

Exercise: Aerobic_____ Strengthening_____

In general, today I feel: Good_____ Fair_____ Poor_____

Pain level (0–10):_____

Drugs/Medications:_____
_____
_____
_____

Vitamins/Herbs:_____
_____
_____
_____

Today's Diet

Breakfast:_____
_____
_____
_____
_____

Lunch:_____
_____
_____
_____

Dinner:_____
_____
_____
_____

Snacks:_____

_____

_____

Thoughts and Feelings Today

_____

_____

_____

_____

_____

_____

_____

_____

_____

_____

_____

_____

_____

_____

_____

_____

_____

_____

_____

_____

_____

_____

_____

_____

_____

ROSEMARY R. KING APRN, BC

Date:_____ Weight:_____ BP:_____

Blood sugar level:_____ Hours slept last night:_____

If using a FitBit or other device, number of steps taken today: _____

Exercise: Aerobic_____ Strengthening_____

In general, today I feel: Good_____ Fair_____ Poor_____

Pain level (0–10):_____

Drugs/Medications:_____

_____

_____

_____

Vitamins/Herbs:_____

_____

_____

_____

Today's Diet

Breakfast:_____

_____

_____

_____

_____

Lunch:_____

_____

_____

_____

Dinner:_____

_____

_____

_____

Snacks:_____

_____

_____

Thoughts and Feelings Today

_____

_____

_____

_____

_____

_____

_____

_____

_____

_____

_____

_____

_____

_____

_____

_____

_____

_____

_____

_____

_____

_____

_____

_____

_____

_____

_____

_____

ROSEMARY R. KING APRN, BC

Date:_____ Weight:_____ BP:_____

Blood sugar level:_____ Hours slept last night:_____

If using a FitBit or other device, number of steps taken today: _____

Exercise: Aerobic_____ Strengthening_____

In general, today I feel: Good_____ Fair_____ Poor_____

Pain level (0–10):_____

Drugs/Medications:_____

_____

_____

_____

Vitamins/Herbs:_____

_____

_____

_____

Today's Diet

Breakfast:_____

_____

_____

_____

Lunch:_____

_____

_____

_____

Dinner:_____

_____

_____

_____

Snacks:_____

_____

_____

Thoughts and Feelings Today

_____

_____

_____

_____

_____

_____

_____

_____

_____

_____

_____

_____

_____

_____

_____

_____

_____

_____

_____

_____

_____

_____

_____

_____

_____

Date:_____Weight:_____BP:_____

Blood sugar level:_____ Hours slept last night:_____

If using a FitBit or other device, number of steps taken today: _____

Exercise: Aerobic_____ Strengthening_____

In general, today I feel: Good_____ Fair_____ Poor_____

Pain level (0–10):_____

Drugs/Medications:_____

_____

_____

_____

Vitamins/Herbs:_____

_____

_____

_____

Today's Diet

Breakfast:_____

_____

_____

_____

Lunch:_____

_____

_____

_____

Dinner:_____

_____

_____

_____

Snacks:_____

_____

_____

Thoughts and Feelings Today

_____

_____

_____

_____

_____

_____

_____

_____

_____

_____

_____

_____

_____

_____

_____

_____

_____

_____

_____

_____

_____

_____

_____

_____

_____

ROSEMARY R. KING APRN, BC

Date:_____Weight:_____BP:_____

Blood sugar level:_____ Hours slept last night:_____

If using a FitBit or other device, number of steps taken today: _____

Exercise: Aerobic_____ Strengthening_____

In general, today I feel: Good_____ Fair_____ Poor_____

Pain level (0–10):_____

Drugs/Medications:_____
_____
_____
_____

Vitamins/Herbs:_____
_____
_____
_____

Today's Diet

Breakfast:_____
_____
_____
_____
_____

Lunch:_____
_____
_____
_____

Dinner:_____
_____
_____
_____

Snacks:_____

_____

_____

Thoughts and Feelings Today

_____

_____

_____

_____

_____

_____

_____

_____

_____

_____

_____

_____

_____

_____

_____

_____

_____

_____

_____

_____

_____

_____

_____

_____

ROSEMARY R. KING APRN, BC

Date:_____ Weight:_____ BP:_____

Blood sugar level:_____ Hours slept last night:_____

If using a FitBit or other device, number of steps taken today: _____

Exercise: Aerobic_____ Strengthening_____

In general, today I feel: Good_____ Fair_____ Poor_____

Pain level (0–10):_____

Drugs/Medications:_____
_____
_____
_____

Vitamins/Herbs:_____
_____
_____
_____

Today's Diet

Breakfast:_____
_____
_____
_____

Lunch:_____
_____
_____
_____

Dinner:_____
_____
_____
_____

Snacks:_____

_____

_____

Thoughts and Feelings Today

_____

_____

_____

_____

_____

_____

_____

_____

_____

_____

_____

_____

_____

_____

_____

_____

_____

_____

_____

_____

_____

_____

_____

_____

_____

_____

_____

Date:_____ Weight:_____ BP:_____

Blood sugar level:_____ Hours slept last night:_____

If using a FitBit or other device, number of steps taken today: _____

Exercise: Aerobic_____ Strengthening_____

In general, today I feel: Good_____ Fair_____ Poor_____

Pain level (0–10):_____

Drugs/Medications:_____
_____
_____
_____

Vitamins/Herbs:_____
_____
_____
_____

Today's Diet

Breakfast:_____
_____
_____
_____

Lunch:_____
_____
_____
_____

Dinner:_____
_____
_____
_____

Snacks:_____

Thoughts and Feelings Today

_____
_____
_____
_____
_____
_____
_____
_____
_____
_____
_____
_____
_____
_____
_____
_____
_____
_____
_____
_____
_____
_____
_____
_____
_____
_____

ROSEMARY R. KING APRN, BC

Date:_____ Weight:_____ BP:_____

Blood sugar level:_____ Hours slept last night:_____

If using a FitBit or other device, number of steps taken today: _____

Exercise: Aerobic_____ Strengthening_____

In general, today I feel: Good_____ Fair_____ Poor_____

Pain level (0–10):_____

Drugs/Medications:_____

_____

_____

_____

Vitamins/Herbs:_____

_____

_____

_____

Today's Diet

Breakfast:_____

_____

_____

_____

_____

Lunch:_____

_____

_____

_____

Dinner:_____

_____

_____

_____

Snacks:_____

_____

_____

Thoughts and Feelings Today

_____

_____

_____

_____

_____

_____

_____

_____

_____

_____

_____

_____

_____

_____

_____

_____

_____

_____

_____

_____

_____

_____

_____

_____

_____

_____

_____

ROSEMARY R. KING APRN, BC

Date:_____Weight:_____BP:_____

Blood sugar level:_____ Hours slept last night:_____

If using a FitBit or other device, number of steps taken today: _____

Exercise: Aerobic_____ Strengthening_____

In general, today I feel: Good_____ Fair_____ Poor_____

Pain level (0–10):_____

Drugs/Medications:_____

_____

_____

_____

Vitamins/Herbs:_____

_____

_____

_____

Today's Diet

Breakfast:_____

_____

_____

_____

_____

Lunch:_____

_____

_____

_____

Dinner:_____

_____

_____

_____

Snacks:_____

_____

_____

Thoughts and Feelings Today

_____

_____

_____

_____

_____

_____

_____

_____

_____

_____

_____

_____

_____

_____

_____

_____

_____

_____

_____

_____

_____

_____

_____

_____

_____

ROSEMARY R. KING APRN, BC

Date:_____Weight:_____BP:_____

Blood sugar level:_____ Hours slept last night:_____

If using a FitBit or other device, number of steps taken today: _____

Exercise: Aerobic_____ Strengthening_____

In general, today I feel: Good_____ Fair_____ Poor_____

Pain level (0–10):_____

Drugs/Medications:_____

_____

_____

_____

Vitamins/Herbs:_____

_____

_____

_____

Today's Diet

Breakfast:_____

_____

_____

_____

Lunch:_____

_____

_____

_____

Dinner:_____

_____

_____

_____

Snacks:_____

_____

Thoughts and Feelings Today

_____
_____
_____
_____
_____
_____
_____
_____
_____
_____
_____
_____
_____
_____
_____
_____
_____
_____
_____
_____
_____
_____
_____
_____
_____
_____

ROSEMARY R. KING APRN, BC

Date:_____Weight:_____BP:_____

Blood sugar level:_____ Hours slept last night:_____

If using a FitBit or other device, number of steps taken today: _____

Exercise: Aerobic_____ Strengthening_____

In general, today I feel: Good_____ Fair_____ Poor_____

Pain level (0–10):_____

Drugs/Medications:_____
_____
_____
_____

Vitamins/Herbs:_____
_____
_____
_____

Today's Diet

Breakfast:_____
_____
_____
_____

Lunch:_____
_____
_____
_____

Dinner:_____
_____
_____
_____

Snacks:_____

_____

_____

Thoughts and Feelings Today

_____

_____

_____

_____

_____

_____

_____

_____

_____

_____

_____

_____

_____

_____

_____

_____

_____

_____

_____

_____

_____

_____

_____

_____

_____

_____

Date:_____Weight:_____BP:_____

Blood sugar level:_____ Hours slept last night:_____

If using a FitBit or other device, number of steps taken today: _____

Exercise: Aerobic_____ Strengthening_____

In general, today I feel: Good_____ Fair_____ Poor_____

Pain level (0–10):_____

Drugs/Medications:_____
_____
_____
_____

Vitamins/Herbs:_____
_____
_____
_____

Today's Diet

Breakfast:_____
_____
_____
_____

Lunch:_____
_____
_____
_____

Dinner:_____
_____
_____
_____

Snacks:_____

_____

_____

Thoughts and Feelings Today

_____

_____

_____

_____

_____

_____

_____

_____

_____

_____

_____

_____

_____

_____

_____

_____

_____

_____

_____

_____

_____

_____

_____

_____

_____

_____

_____

_____

ROSEMARY R. KING APRN, BC

Date:_____Weight:_____BP:_____

Blood sugar level:_____ Hours slept last night:_____

If using a FitBit or other device, number of steps taken today: _____

Exercise: Aerobic_____ Strengthening_____

In general, today I feel: Good_____ Fair_____ Poor_____

Pain level (0–10):_____

Drugs/Medications:_____
_____
_____
_____

Vitamins/Herbs:_____
_____
_____
_____

Today's Diet

Breakfast:_____
_____
_____
_____

Lunch:_____
_____
_____
_____

Dinner:_____
_____
_____
_____

Snacks:_____

_____

Thoughts and Feelings Today

_____
_____
_____
_____
_____
_____
_____
_____
_____
_____
_____
_____
_____
_____
_____
_____
_____
_____
_____
_____
_____
_____
_____
_____

Date:_____Weight:_____BP:_____

Blood sugar level:_____ Hours slept last night:_____

If using a FitBit or other device, number of steps taken today: _____

Exercise: Aerobic_____ Strengthening_____

In general, today I feel: Good_____ Fair_____ Poor_____

Pain level (0–10):_____

Drugs/Medications:_____

_____

_____

_____

Vitamins/Herbs:_____

_____

_____

_____

Today's Diet

Breakfast:_____

_____

_____

_____

_____

Lunch:_____

_____

_____

_____

Dinner:_____

_____

_____

_____

Snacks:_____

_____

Thoughts and Feelings Today

_____

_____

_____

_____

_____

_____

_____

_____

_____

_____

_____

_____

_____

_____

_____

_____

_____

_____

_____

_____

_____

_____

_____

_____

_____

_____

_____

ROSEMARY R. KING APRN, BC

Date:_____Weight:_____BP:_____

Blood sugar level:_____ Hours slept last night:_____

If using a FitBit or other device, number of steps taken today: _____

Exercise: Aerobic_____ Strengthening_____

In general, today I feel: Good_____ Fair_____ Poor_____

Pain level (0–10):_____

Drugs/Medications:_____
_____
_____
_____

Vitamins/Herbs:_____
_____
_____
_____

Today's Diet

Breakfast:_____
_____
_____
_____

Lunch:_____
_____
_____

Dinner:_____
_____
_____
_____

Snacks:_____

_____

_____

Thoughts and Feelings Today

_____

_____

_____

_____

_____

_____

_____

_____

_____

_____

_____

_____

_____

_____

_____

_____

_____

_____

_____

_____

_____

_____

_____

_____

_____

_____

_____

ROSEMARY R. KING APRN, BC

Date:_____ Weight:_____ BP:_____

Blood sugar level:_____ Hours slept last night:_____

If using a FitBit or other device, number of steps taken today: _____

Exercise: Aerobic_____ Strengthening_____

In general, today I feel: Good_____ Fair_____ Poor_____

Pain level (0–10):_____

Drugs/Medications:_____

_____

_____

_____

Vitamins/Herbs:_____

_____

_____

_____

Today's Diet

Breakfast:_____

_____

_____

_____

_____

Lunch:_____

_____

_____

_____

Dinner:_____

_____

_____

_____

Snacks:_____
_____

Thoughts and Feelings Today

_____
_____
_____
_____
_____
_____
_____
_____
_____
_____
_____
_____
_____
_____
_____
_____
_____
_____
_____
_____
_____
_____
_____
_____
_____
_____
_____

ROSEMARY R. KING APRN, BC

Date:_____Weight:_____BP:_____

Blood sugar level:_____ Hours slept last night:_____

If using a FitBit or other device, number of steps taken today: _____

Exercise: Aerobic_____ Strengthening_____

In general, today I feel: Good_____ Fair_____ Poor_____

Pain level (0–10):_____

Drugs/Medications:_____
_____
_____
_____

Vitamins/Herbs:_____
_____
_____
_____

Today's Diet

Breakfast:_____
_____
_____
_____

Lunch:_____
_____
_____
_____

Dinner:_____
_____
_____
_____

Snacks:_____

_____

Thoughts and Feelings Today

_____

_____

_____

_____

_____

_____

_____

_____

_____

_____

_____

_____

_____

_____

_____

_____

_____

_____

_____

_____

_____

_____

_____

_____

ROSEMARY R. KING APRN, BC

Date:_____ Weight:_____ BP:_____

Blood sugar level:_____ Hours slept last night:_____

If using a FitBit or other device, number of steps taken today: _____

Exercise: Aerobic_____ Strengthening_____

In general, today I feel: Good_____ Fair_____ Poor_____

Pain level (0–10):_____

Drugs/Medications:_____

_____

_____

_____

Vitamins/Herbs:_____

_____

_____

_____

Today's Diet

Breakfast:_____

_____

_____

_____

Lunch:_____

_____

_____

_____

Dinner:_____

_____

_____

_____

Snacks:_____

_____

_____

Thoughts and Feelings Today

_____
_____
_____
_____
_____
_____
_____
_____
_____
_____
_____
_____
_____
_____
_____
_____
_____
_____
_____
_____
_____
_____
_____
_____
_____
_____
_____

Date:_____Weight:_____BP:_____

Blood sugar level:_____ Hours slept last night:_____

If using a FitBit or other device, number of steps taken today: _____

Exercise: Aerobic_____ Strengthening_____

In general, today I feel: Good_____ Fair_____ Poor_____

Pain level (0–10):_____

Drugs/Medications:_____
_____
_____
_____

Vitamins/Herbs:_____
_____
_____
_____

Today's Diet

Breakfast:_____
_____
_____
_____
_____

Lunch:_____
_____
_____
_____

Dinner:_____
_____
_____
_____

Snacks:_____

_____

Thoughts and Feelings Today

_____
_____
_____
_____
_____
_____
_____
_____
_____
_____
_____
_____
_____
_____
_____
_____
_____
_____
_____
_____
_____
_____
_____
_____

ROSEMARY R. KING APRN, BC

Date:_____Weight:_____BP:_____

Blood sugar level:_____ Hours slept last night:_____

If using a FitBit or other device, number of steps taken today: _____

Exercise: Aerobic_____ Strengthening_____

In general, today I feel: Good_____ Fair_____ Poor_____

Pain level (0–10):_____

Drugs/Medications:_____

_____

_____

_____

Vitamins/Herbs:_____

_____

_____

_____

Today's Diet

Breakfast:_____

_____

_____

_____

Lunch:_____

_____

_____

_____

Dinner:_____

_____

_____

_____

Snacks:_____

_____

Thoughts and Feelings Today

_____

_____

_____

_____

_____

_____

_____

_____

_____

_____

_____

_____

_____

_____

_____

_____

_____

_____

_____

_____

_____

_____

_____

_____

_____

_____

_____

Date:_____Weight:_____BP:_____

Blood sugar level:_____ Hours slept last night:_____

If using a FitBit or other device, number of steps taken today: _____

Exercise: Aerobic_____ Strengthening_____

In general, today I feel: Good_____ Fair_____ Poor_____

Pain level (0–10):_____

Drugs/Medications:_____
_____
_____
_____

Vitamins/Herbs:_____
_____
_____
_____

Today's Diet

Breakfast:_____
_____
_____
_____

Lunch:_____
_____
_____
_____

Dinner:_____
_____
_____
_____

Snacks:_____

_____

_____

Thoughts and Feelings Today

_____

_____

_____

_____

_____

_____

_____

_____

_____

_____

_____

_____

_____

_____

_____

_____

_____

_____

_____

_____

_____

_____

_____

Date:_____Weight:_____BP:_____

Blood sugar level:_____ Hours slept last night:_____

If using a FitBit or other device, number of steps taken today: _____

Exercise: Aerobic_____ Strengthening_____

In general, today I feel: Good_____ Fair_____ Poor_____

Pain level (0–10):_____

Drugs/Medications:_____
_____
_____
_____

Vitamins/Herbs:_____
_____
_____
_____

Today's Diet

Breakfast:_____
_____
_____
_____
_____

Lunch:_____
_____
_____
_____

Dinner:_____
_____
_____
_____

Snacks:_____

_____

Thoughts and Feelings Today

_____

_____

_____

_____

_____

_____

_____

_____

_____

_____

_____

_____

_____

_____

_____

_____

_____

_____

_____

_____

_____

_____

_____

_____

ROSEMARY R. KING APRN, BC

Date:_____Weight:_____BP:_____

Blood sugar level:_____ Hours slept last night:_____

If using a FitBit or other device, number of steps taken today: _____

Exercise: Aerobic_____ Strengthening_____

In general, today I feel: Good_____ Fair_____ Poor_____

Pain level (0–10):_____

Drugs/Medications:_____

_____

_____

_____

Vitamins/Herbs:_____

_____

_____

_____

Today's Diet

Breakfast:_____

_____

_____

_____

_____

Lunch:_____

_____

_____

_____

Dinner:_____

_____

_____

_____

Snacks:_____

_____

_____

Thoughts and Feelings Today

_____

_____

_____

_____

_____

_____

_____

_____

_____

_____

_____

_____

_____

_____

_____

_____

_____

_____

_____

_____

_____

_____

_____

_____

ROSEMARY R. KING APRN, BC

Date:_____Weight:_____BP:_____

Blood sugar level:_____ Hours slept last night:_____

If using a FitBit or other device, number of steps taken today: _____

Exercise: Aerobic_____ Strengthening_____

In general, today I feel: Good_____ Fair_____ Poor_____

Pain level (0–10):_____

Drugs/Medications:_____
_____
_____
_____

Vitamins/Herbs:_____
_____
_____
_____

Today's Diet

Breakfast:_____
_____
_____
_____
_____

Lunch:_____
_____
_____
_____

Dinner:_____
_____
_____
_____

Snacks:_____

_____

Thoughts and Feelings Today

_____

_____

_____

_____

_____

_____

_____

_____

_____

_____

_____

_____

_____

_____

_____

_____

_____

_____

_____

_____

_____

_____

_____

_____

ROSEMARY R. KING APRN, BC

Date:_____ Weight:_____ BP:_____

Blood sugar level:_____ Hours slept last night:_____

If using a FitBit or other device, number of steps taken today: _____

Exercise: Aerobic_____ Strengthening_____

In general, today I feel: Good_____ Fair_____ Poor_____

Pain level (0–10):_____

Drugs/Medications:_____
_____
_____
_____

Vitamins/Herbs:_____
_____
_____
_____

Today's Diet

Breakfast:_____
_____
_____
_____
_____

Lunch:_____
_____
_____
_____

Dinner:_____
_____
_____
_____

Snacks:_____

_____

_____

Thoughts and Feelings Today

_____

_____

_____

_____

_____

_____

_____

_____

_____

_____

_____

_____

_____

_____

_____

_____

_____

_____

_____

_____

_____

_____

_____

_____

ROSEMARY R. KING APRN, BC

Date:_____Weight:_____BP:_____

Blood sugar level:_____ Hours slept last night:_____

If using a FitBit or other device, number of steps taken today: _____

Exercise: Aerobic_____ Strengthening_____

In general, today I feel: Good_____ Fair_____ Poor_____

Pain level (0–10):_____

Drugs/Medications:_____
_____
_____
_____

Vitamins/Herbs:_____
_____
_____
_____

Today's Diet

Breakfast:_____
_____
_____
_____
_____

Lunch:_____
_____
_____
_____

Dinner:_____
_____
_____
_____

Snacks:_____

_____

Thoughts and Feelings Today

_____
_____
_____
_____
_____
_____
_____
_____
_____
_____
_____
_____
_____
_____
_____
_____
_____
_____
_____
_____
_____
_____
_____
_____
_____

ROSEMARY R. KING APRN, BC

Date:_____Weight:_____BP:_____

Blood sugar level:_____ Hours slept last night:_____

If using a FitBit or other device, number of steps taken today: _____

Exercise: Aerobic_____ Strengthening_____

In general, today I feel: Good_____ Fair_____ Poor_____

Pain level (0–10):_____

Drugs/Medications:_____

_____

_____

_____

Vitamins/Herbs:_____

_____

_____

_____

Today's Diet

Breakfast:_____

_____

_____

_____

_____

Lunch:_____

_____

_____

_____

Dinner:_____

_____

_____

_____

Snacks:_____

_____

_____

Thoughts and Feelings Today

_____

_____

_____

_____

_____

_____

_____

_____

_____

_____

_____

_____

_____

_____

_____

_____

_____

_____

_____

_____

_____

_____

_____

ROSEMARY R. KING APRN, BC

Date:_____Weight:_____BP:_____

Blood sugar level:_____ Hours slept last night:_____

If using a FitBit or other device, number of steps taken today: _____

Exercise: Aerobic_____ Strengthening_____

In general, today I feel: Good_____ Fair_____ Poor_____

Pain level (0–10):_____

Drugs/Medications:_____

_____

_____

_____

Vitamins/Herbs:_____

_____

_____

_____

Today's Diet

Breakfast:_____

_____

_____

_____

_____

Lunch:_____

_____

_____

_____

Dinner:_____

_____

_____

_____

Snacks:_____

_____

_____

Thoughts and Feelings Today

_____
_____
_____
_____
_____
_____
_____
_____
_____
_____
_____
_____
_____
_____
_____
_____
_____
_____
_____
_____
_____
_____
_____
_____
_____

ROSEMARY R. KING APRN, BC

Date:_____Weight:_____BP:_____

Blood sugar level:_____ Hours slept last night:_____

If using a FitBit or other device, number of steps taken today: _____

Exercise: Aerobic_____ Strengthening_____

In general, today I feel: Good_____ Fair_____ Poor_____

Pain level (0–10):_____

Drugs/Medications:_____

_____

_____

_____

Vitamins/Herbs:_____

_____

_____

_____

Today's Diet

Breakfast:_____

_____

_____

_____

Lunch:_____

_____

_____

_____

Dinner:_____

_____

_____

_____

Snacks:_____

_____

_____

Thoughts and Feelings Today

_____

_____

_____

_____

_____

_____

_____

_____

_____

_____

_____

_____

_____

_____

_____

_____

_____

_____

_____

_____

_____

_____

_____

_____

_____

ROSEMARY R. KING APRN, BC

Date:_____ Weight:_____ BP:_____

Blood sugar level:_____ Hours slept last night:_____

If using a FitBit or other device, number of steps taken today: _____

Exercise: Aerobic_____ Strengthening_____

In general, today I feel: Good_____ Fair_____ Poor_____

Pain level (0–10):_____

Drugs/Medications:_____
_____
_____
_____

Vitamins/Herbs:_____
_____
_____
_____

Today's Diet

Breakfast:_____
_____
_____
_____
_____

Lunch:_____
_____
_____
_____

Dinner:_____
_____
_____
_____

Snacks:_____

_____

_____

Thoughts and Feelings Today

_____

_____

_____

_____

_____

_____

_____

_____

_____

_____

_____

_____

_____

_____

_____

_____

_____

_____

_____

_____

_____

_____

_____

_____

_____

_____

_____

ROSEMARY R. KING APRN, BC

Date:_____ Weight:_____ BP:_____

Blood sugar level:_____ Hours slept last night:_____

If using a FitBit or other device, number of steps taken today: _____

Exercise: Aerobic_____ Strengthening_____

In general, today I feel: Good_____ Fair_____ Poor_____

Pain level (0–10):_____

Drugs/Medications:_____

_____

_____

_____

Vitamins/Herbs:_____

_____

_____

_____

Today's Diet

Breakfast:_____

_____

_____

_____

_____

Lunch:_____

_____

_____

_____

Dinner:_____

_____

_____

_____

Snacks:_____

_____

_____

Thoughts and Feelings Today

_____

_____

_____

_____

_____

_____

_____

_____

_____

_____

_____

_____

_____

_____

_____

_____

_____

_____

_____

_____

_____

_____

_____

_____

_____

_____

ROSEMARY R. KING APRN, BC

Date:_____ Weight:_____ BP:_____

Blood sugar level:_____ Hours slept last night:_____

If using a FitBit or other device, number of steps taken today: _____

Exercise: Aerobic_____ Strengthening_____

In general, today I feel: Good_____ Fair_____ Poor_____

Pain level (0–10):_____

Drugs/Medications:_____

_____

_____

_____

Vitamins/Herbs:_____

_____

_____

_____

Today's Diet

Breakfast:_____

_____

_____

_____

_____

Lunch:_____

_____

_____

_____

Dinner:_____

_____

_____

_____

Snacks:_____

_____

_____

Thoughts and Feelings Today

_____
_____
_____
_____
_____
_____
_____
_____
_____
_____
_____
_____
_____
_____
_____
_____
_____
_____
_____
_____
_____
_____
_____
_____

ROSEMARY R. KING APRN, BC

Date:_____ Weight:_____ BP:_____

Blood sugar level:_____ Hours slept last night:_____

If using a FitBit or other device, number of steps taken today: _____

Exercise: Aerobic_____ Strengthening_____

In general, today I feel: Good_____ Fair_____ Poor_____

Pain level (0–10):_____

Drugs/Medications:_____

_____

_____

_____

Vitamins/Herbs:_____

_____

_____

_____

Today's Diet

Breakfast:_____

_____

_____

_____

_____

Lunch:_____

_____

_____

_____

Dinner:_____

_____

_____

_____

Snacks:_____

_____

_____

Thoughts and Feelings Today

_____

_____

_____

_____

_____

_____

_____

_____

_____

_____

_____

_____

_____

_____

_____

_____

_____

_____

_____

_____

_____

_____

_____

_____

_____

ROSEMARY R. KING APRN, BC

Date:_____Weight:_____BP:_____

Blood sugar level:_____ Hours slept last night:_____

If using a FitBit or other device, number of steps taken today: _____

Exercise: Aerobic_____ Strengthening_____

In general, today I feel: Good_____ Fair_____ Poor_____

Pain level (0–10):_____

Drugs/Medications:_____
_____
_____
_____

Vitamins/Herbs:_____
_____
_____
_____

Today's Diet

Breakfast:_____
_____
_____
_____
_____

Lunch:_____
_____
_____
_____

Dinner:_____
_____
_____
_____

Snacks:_____

_____

_____

Thoughts and Feelings Today

_____

_____

_____

_____

_____

_____

_____

_____

_____

_____

_____

_____

_____

_____

_____

_____

_____

_____

_____

_____

_____

_____

_____

ROSEMARY R. KING APRN, BC

Date:_____Weight:_____BP:_____

Blood sugar level:_____ Hours slept last night:_____

If using a FitBit or other device, number of steps taken today: _____

Exercise: Aerobic_____ Strengthening_____

In general, today I feel: Good_____ Fair_____ Poor_____

Pain level (0–10):_____

Drugs/Medications:_____
_____
_____
_____

Vitamins/Herbs:_____
_____
_____
_____

Today's Diet

Breakfast:_____
_____
_____
_____

Lunch:_____
_____
_____

Dinner:_____
_____
_____

Snacks:_____

_____

Thoughts and Feelings Today

_____

_____

_____

_____

_____

_____

_____

_____

_____

_____

_____

_____

_____

_____

_____

_____

_____

_____

_____

_____

_____

_____

_____

_____

_____

Date:_____Weight:_____BP:_____

Blood sugar level:_____ Hours slept last night:_____

If using a FitBit or other device, number of steps taken today: _____

Exercise: Aerobic_____ Strengthening_____

In general, today I feel: Good_____ Fair_____ Poor_____

Pain level (0–10):_____

Drugs/Medications:_____
_____
_____
_____

Vitamins/Herbs:_____
_____
_____
_____

Today's Diet

Breakfast:_____
_____
_____
_____

Lunch:_____
_____
_____
_____

Dinner:_____
_____
_____
_____

Snacks:_____

_____

_____

Thoughts and Feelings Today

_____

_____

_____

_____

_____

_____

_____

_____

_____

_____

_____

_____

_____

_____

_____

_____

_____

_____

_____

_____

_____

_____

_____

_____

Date:_____Weight:_____BP:_____

Blood sugar level:_____ Hours slept last night:_____

If using a FitBit or other device, number of steps taken today: _____

Exercise: Aerobic_____ Strengthening_____

In general, today I feel: Good_____ Fair_____ Poor_____

Pain level (0–10):_____

Drugs/Medications:_____

_____

_____

_____

Vitamins/Herbs:_____

_____

_____

_____

Today's Diet

Breakfast:_____

_____

_____

_____

Lunch:_____

_____

_____

_____

Dinner:_____

_____

_____

_____

Snacks:_____

_____

_____

Thoughts and Feelings Today

_____

_____

_____

_____

_____

_____

_____

_____

_____

_____

_____

_____

_____

_____

_____

_____

_____

_____

_____

_____

_____

_____

_____

ROSEMARY R. KING APRN, BC

Date:_____Weight:_____BP:_____

Blood sugar level:_____ Hours slept last night:_____

If using a FitBit or other device, number of steps taken today: _____

Exercise: Aerobic_____ Strengthening_____

In general, today I feel: Good_____ Fair_____ Poor_____

Pain level (0–10):_____

Drugs/Medications:_____

_____

_____

_____

Vitamins/Herbs:_____

_____

_____

_____

Today's Diet

Breakfast:_____

_____

_____

_____

_____

Lunch:_____

_____

_____

_____

Dinner:_____

_____

_____

_____

Snacks:_____

_____

_____

Thoughts and Feelings Today

_____

_____

_____

_____

_____

_____

_____

_____

_____

_____

_____

_____

_____

_____

_____

_____

_____

_____

_____

_____

_____

_____

_____

_____

_____

ROSEMARY R. KING APRN, BC

Date:_____Weight:_____BP:_____

Blood sugar level:_____ Hours slept last night:_____

If using a FitBit or other device, number of steps taken today: _____

Exercise: Aerobic_____ Strengthening_____

In general, today I feel: Good_____ Fair_____ Poor_____

Pain level (0–10):_____

Drugs/Medications:_____
_____
_____
_____

Vitamins/Herbs:_____
_____
_____
_____

Today's Diet

Breakfast:_____
_____
_____
_____
_____

Lunch:_____
_____
_____
_____

Dinner:_____
_____
_____
_____

Snacks:_____

_____

Thoughts and Feelings Today

_____

_____

_____

_____

_____

_____

_____

_____

_____

_____

_____

_____

_____

_____

_____

_____

_____

_____

_____

_____

_____

ROSEMARY R. KING APRN, BC

Date:_____Weight:_____BP:_____

Blood sugar level:_____ Hours slept last night:_____

If using a FitBit or other device, number of steps taken today: _____

Exercise: Aerobic_____ Strengthening_____

In general, today I feel: Good_____ Fair_____ Poor_____

Pain level (0–10):_____

Drugs/Medications:_____

_____

_____

_____

Vitamins/Herbs:_____

_____

_____

_____

Today's Diet

Breakfast:_____

_____

_____

_____

_____

Lunch:_____

_____

_____

_____

Dinner:_____

_____

_____

_____

Snacks:_____

_____

_____

Thoughts and Feelings Today

_____

_____

_____

_____

_____

_____

_____

_____

_____

_____

_____

_____

_____

_____

_____

_____

_____

_____

_____

_____

_____

_____

_____

_____

_____

_____

_____

Date:_____Weight:_____BP:_____

Blood sugar level:_____ Hours slept last night:_____

If using a FitBit or other device, number of steps taken today: _____

Exercise: Aerobic_____ Strengthening_____

In general, today I feel: Good_____ Fair_____ Poor_____

Pain level (0–10):_____

Drugs/Medications:_____

_____

_____

_____

Vitamins/Herbs:_____

_____

_____

_____

Today's Diet

Breakfast:_____

_____

_____

_____

_____

Lunch:_____

_____

_____

_____

Dinner:_____

_____

_____

_____

Snacks:_____

_____

Thoughts and Feelings Today

_____

_____

_____

_____

_____

_____

_____

_____

_____

_____

_____

_____

_____

_____

_____

_____

_____

_____

_____

_____

_____

_____

_____

_____

_____

_____

Date:_____Weight:_____BP:_____

Blood sugar level:_____ Hours slept last night:_____

If using a FitBit or other device, number of steps taken today: _____

Exercise: Aerobic_____ Strengthening_____

In general, today I feel: Good_____ Fair_____ Poor_____

Pain level (0–10):_____

Drugs/Medications:_____

_____

_____

_____

Vitamins/Herbs:_____

_____

_____

_____

Today's Diet

Breakfast:_____

_____

_____

_____

_____

Lunch:_____

_____

_____

_____

Dinner:_____

_____

_____

_____

Snacks:_____

_____

_____

Thoughts and Feelings Today

_____

_____

_____

_____

_____

_____

_____

_____

_____

_____

_____

_____

_____

_____

_____

_____

_____

_____

_____

_____

_____

_____

_____

ROSEMARY R. KING APRN, BC

Date:_____Weight:_____BP:_____

Blood sugar level:_____ Hours slept last night:_____

If using a FitBit or other device, number of steps taken today: _____

Exercise: Aerobic_____ Strengthening_____

In general, today I feel: Good_____ Fair_____ Poor_____

Pain level (0–10):_____

Drugs/Medications:_____
_____
_____
_____

Vitamins/Herbs:_____
_____
_____
_____

Today's Diet

Breakfast:_____
_____
_____
_____
_____

Lunch:_____
_____
_____
_____

Dinner:_____
_____
_____
_____

Snacks:_____

_____

_____

Thoughts and Feelings Today

_____

_____

_____

_____

_____

_____

_____

_____

_____

_____

_____

_____

_____

_____

_____

_____

_____

_____

_____

_____

_____

_____

ROSEMARY R. KING APRN, BC

Date:_____Weight:_____BP:_____

Blood sugar level:_____ Hours slept last night:_____

If using a FitBit or other device, number of steps taken today: _____

Exercise: Aerobic_____ Strengthening_____

In general, today I feel: Good_____ Fair_____ Poor_____

Pain level (0–10):_____

Drugs/Medications:_____

_____

_____

_____

Vitamins/Herbs:_____

_____

_____

_____

Today's Diet

Breakfast:_____

_____

_____

_____

_____

Lunch:_____

_____

_____

_____

Dinner:_____

_____

_____

_____

Snacks:_____

Thoughts and Feelings Today

_____

_____

_____

_____

_____

_____

_____

_____

_____

_____

_____

_____

_____

_____

_____

_____

_____

_____

_____

_____

_____

_____

_____

_____

ROSEMARY R. KING APRN, BC

Date:_____Weight:_____BP:_____

Blood sugar level:_____ Hours slept last night:_____

If using a FitBit or other device, number of steps taken today: _____

Exercise: Aerobic_____ Strengthening_____

In general, today I feel: Good_____ Fair_____ Poor_____

Pain level (0–10):_____

Drugs/Medications:_____
_____
_____
_____

Vitamins/Herbs:_____
_____
_____
_____

Today's Diet

Breakfast:_____
_____
_____
_____

Lunch:_____
_____
_____
_____

Dinner:_____
_____
_____
_____

Snacks:_____

_____

_____

Thoughts and Feelings Today

_____

_____

_____

_____

_____

_____

_____

_____

_____

_____

_____

_____

_____

_____

_____

_____

_____

_____

_____

_____

_____

_____

_____

_____

_____

ROSEMARY R. KING APRN, BC

Date:_____ Weight:_____ BP:_____

Blood sugar level:_____ Hours slept last night:_____

If using a FitBit or other device, number of steps taken today: _____

Exercise: Aerobic_____ Strengthening_____

In general, today I feel: Good_____ Fair_____ Poor_____

Pain level (0–10):_____

Drugs/Medications:_____
_____
_____
_____

Vitamins/Herbs:_____
_____
_____
_____

Today's Diet

Breakfast:_____
_____
_____
_____
_____

Lunch:_____
_____
_____
_____

Dinner:_____
_____
_____
_____

Snacks:_____

_____

_____

Thoughts and Feelings Today

_____

_____

_____

_____

_____

_____

_____

_____

_____

_____

_____

_____

_____

_____

_____

_____

_____

_____

_____

_____

_____

_____

_____

_____

_____

_____

ROSEMARY R. KING APRN, BC

Date:_____Weight:_____BP:_____

Blood sugar level:_____ Hours slept last night:_____

If using a FitBit or other device, number of steps taken today: _____

Exercise: Aerobic_____ Strengthening_____

In general, today I feel: Good_____ Fair_____ Poor_____

Pain level (0–10):_____

Drugs/Medications:_____
_____
_____
_____

Vitamins/Herbs:_____
_____
_____
_____

Today's Diet

Breakfast:_____
_____
_____
_____
_____

Lunch:_____
_____
_____
_____
_____

Dinner:_____
_____
_____
_____

Snacks:_____
_____
_____

Thoughts and Feelings Today

_____
_____
_____
_____
_____
_____
_____
_____
_____
_____
_____
_____
_____
_____
_____
_____
_____
_____
_____
_____
_____
_____
_____

ROSEMARY R. KING APRN, BC

Date:_____Weight:_____BP:_____

Blood sugar level:_____ Hours slept last night:_____

If using a FitBit or other device, number of steps taken today: _____

Exercise: Aerobic_____ Strengthening_____

In general, today I feel: Good_____ Fair_____ Poor_____

Pain level (0–10):_____

Drugs/Medications:_____

_____

_____

_____

Vitamins/Herbs:_____

_____

_____

_____

Today's Diet

Breakfast:_____

_____

_____

_____

_____

Lunch:_____

_____

_____

_____

Dinner:_____

_____

_____

_____

Snacks:_____

_____

_____

Thoughts and Feelings Today

_____

_____

_____

_____

_____

_____

_____

_____

_____

_____

_____

_____

_____

_____

_____

_____

_____

_____

_____

_____

_____

_____

_____

_____

_____

ROSEMARY R. KING APRN, BC

Date:_____Weight:_____BP:_____

Blood sugar level:_____ Hours slept last night:_____

If using a FitBit or other device, number of steps taken today: _____

Exercise: Aerobic_____ Strengthening_____

In general, today I feel: Good_____ Fair_____ Poor_____

Pain level (0–10):_____

Drugs/Medications:_____

_____

_____

_____

Vitamins/Herbs:_____

_____

_____

_____

Today's Diet

Breakfast:_____

_____

_____

_____

_____

Lunch:_____

_____

_____

_____

Dinner:_____

_____

_____

_____

Snacks:_____

_____

_____

Thoughts and Feelings Today

_____

_____

_____

_____

_____

_____

_____

_____

_____

_____

_____

_____

_____

_____

_____

_____

_____

_____

_____

_____

_____

_____

_____

ROSEMARY R. KING APRN, BC

Date:_____Weight:_____BP:_____

Blood sugar level:_____ Hours slept last night:_____

If using a FitBit or other device, number of steps taken today: _____

Exercise: Aerobic_____ Strengthening_____

In general, today I feel: Good_____ Fair_____ Poor_____

Pain level (0–10):_____

Drugs/Medications:_____

_____

_____

_____

Vitamins/Herbs:_____

_____

_____

_____

Today's Diet

Breakfast:_____

_____

_____

_____

_____

Lunch:_____

_____

_____

_____

Dinner:_____

_____

_____

_____

Snacks:_____
_____
_____

Thoughts and Feelings Today

_____
_____
_____
_____
_____
_____
_____
_____
_____
_____
_____
_____
_____
_____
_____
_____
_____
_____
_____
_____
_____
_____
_____
_____

ROSEMARY R. KING APRN, BC

Date:_____ Weight:_____ BP:_____

Blood sugar level:_____ Hours slept last night:_____

If using a FitBit or other device, number of steps taken today: _____

Exercise: Aerobic_____ Strengthening_____

In general, today I feel: Good_____ Fair_____ Poor_____

Pain level (0–10):_____

Drugs/Medications:_____

_____

_____

_____

Vitamins/Herbs:_____

_____

_____

_____

Today's Diet

Breakfast:_____

_____

_____

_____

_____

Lunch:_____

_____

_____

_____

Dinner:_____

_____

_____

_____

Snacks:_____

_____

_____

Thoughts and Feelings Today

_____

_____

_____

_____

_____

_____

_____

_____

_____

_____

_____

_____

_____

_____

_____

_____

_____

_____

_____

_____

_____

_____

_____

Date:_____Weight:_____BP:_____

Blood sugar level:_____ Hours slept last night:_____

If using a FitBit or other device, number of steps taken today: _____

Exercise: Aerobic_____ Strengthening_____

In general, today I feel: Good_____ Fair_____ Poor_____

Pain level (0–10):_____

Drugs/Medications:_____
_____
_____
_____

Vitamins/Herbs:_____
_____
_____
_____

Today's Diet

Breakfast:_____
_____
_____
_____
_____

Lunch:_____
_____
_____
_____

Dinner:_____
_____
_____
_____

Snacks:_____

_____

_____

Thoughts and Feelings Today

_____
_____
_____
_____
_____
_____
_____
_____
_____
_____
_____
_____
_____
_____
_____
_____
_____
_____
_____
_____
_____
_____
_____
_____
_____
_____

ROSEMARY R. KING APRN, BC

Date:_____ Weight:_____ BP:_____

Blood sugar level:_____ Hours slept last night:_____

If using a FitBit or other device, number of steps taken today: _____

Exercise: Aerobic_____ Strengthening_____

In general, today I feel: Good_____ Fair_____ Poor_____

Pain level (0–10):_____

Drugs/Medications:_____

_____

_____

_____

Vitamins/Herbs:_____

_____

_____

_____

Today's Diet

Breakfast:_____

_____

_____

_____

_____

Lunch:_____

_____

_____

_____

Dinner:_____

_____

_____

_____

Snacks:_____

_____

_____

Thoughts and Feelings Today

_____

_____

_____

_____

_____

_____

_____

_____

_____

_____

_____

_____

_____

_____

_____

_____

_____

_____

_____

_____

_____

_____

_____

_____

ROSEMARY R. KING APRN, BC

Date:_____Weight:_____BP:_____

Blood sugar level:_____ Hours slept last night:_____

If using a FitBit or other device, number of steps taken today: _____

Exercise: Aerobic_____ Strengthening_____

In general, today I feel: Good_____ Fair_____ Poor_____

Pain level (0–10):_____

Drugs/Medications:_____

_____

_____

_____

_____

Vitamins/Herbs:_____

_____

_____

_____

Today's Diet

Breakfast:_____

_____

_____

_____

_____

Lunch:_____

_____

_____

_____

Dinner:_____

_____

_____

_____

Snacks:_____

_____

_____

Thoughts and Feelings Today

_____

_____

_____

_____

_____

_____

_____

_____

_____

_____

_____

_____

_____

_____

_____

_____

_____

_____

_____

_____

_____

_____

_____

_____

ROSEMARY R. KING APRN, BC

Date:_____ Weight:_____ BP:_____

Blood sugar level:_____ Hours slept last night:_____

If using a FitBit or other device, number of steps taken today: _____

Exercise: Aerobic_____ Strengthening_____

In general, today I feel: Good_____ Fair_____ Poor_____

Pain level (0–10):_____

Drugs/Medications:_____

_____

_____

_____

Vitamins/Herbs:_____

_____

_____

_____

Today's Diet

Breakfast:_____

_____

_____

_____

Lunch:_____

_____

_____

_____

Dinner:_____

_____

_____

_____

Snacks:_____

_____

Thoughts and Feelings Today

_____

_____

_____

_____

_____

_____

_____

_____

_____

_____

_____

_____

_____

_____

_____

_____

_____

_____

_____

_____

_____

_____

_____

_____

ROSEMARY R. KING APRN, BC

Date:_____Weight:_____BP:_____

Blood sugar level:_____ Hours slept last night:_____

If using a FitBit or other device, number of steps taken today: _____

Exercise: Aerobic_____ Strengthening_____

In general, today I feel: Good_____ Fair_____ Poor_____

Pain level (0–10):_____

Drugs/Medications:_____
_____
_____
_____

Vitamins/Herbs:_____
_____
_____
_____

Today's Diet

Breakfast:_____
_____
_____
_____
_____

Lunch:_____
_____
_____
_____

Dinner:_____
_____
_____
_____

Snacks:_____

_____

Thoughts and Feelings Today

_____

_____

_____

_____

_____

_____

_____

_____

_____

_____

_____

_____

_____

_____

_____

_____

_____

_____

_____

_____

_____

_____

_____

ROSEMARY R. KING APRN, BC

Date:_____ Weight:_____ BP:_____

Blood sugar level:_____ Hours slept last night:_____

If using a FitBit or other device, number of steps taken today: _____

Exercise: Aerobic_____ Strengthening_____

In general, today I feel: Good_____ Fair_____ Poor_____

Pain level (0–10):_____

Drugs/Medications:_____

_____

_____

_____

Vitamins/Herbs:_____

_____

_____

_____

Today's Diet

Breakfast:_____

_____

_____

_____

_____

Lunch:_____

_____

_____

_____

Dinner:_____

_____

_____

_____

Snacks:_____

_____

_____

Thoughts and Feelings Today

_____

_____

_____

_____

_____

_____

_____

_____

_____

_____

_____

_____

_____

_____

_____

_____

_____

_____

_____

_____

_____

_____

ROSEMARY R. KING APRN, BC

Date:_____Weight:_____BP:_____

Blood sugar level:_____ Hours slept last night:_____

If using a FitBit or other device, number of steps taken today: _____

Exercise: Aerobic_____ Strengthening_____

In general, today I feel: Good_____ Fair_____ Poor_____

Pain level (0–10):_____

Drugs/Medications:_____

_____

_____

_____

Vitamins/Herbs:_____

_____

_____

_____

Today's Diet

Breakfast:_____

_____

_____

_____

_____

Lunch:_____

_____

_____

_____

Dinner:_____

_____

_____

_____

Snacks:_____

_____

_____

Thoughts and Feelings Today

_____

_____

_____

_____

_____

_____

_____

_____

_____

_____

_____

_____

_____

_____

_____

_____

_____

_____

_____

_____

_____

ROSEMARY R. KING APRN, BC

Date:_____Weight:_____BP:_____

Blood sugar level:_____ Hours slept last night:_____

If using a FitBit or other device, number of steps taken today: _____

Exercise: Aerobic_____ Strengthening_____

In general, today I feel: Good_____ Fair_____ Poor_____

Pain level (0–10):_____

Drugs/Medications:_____

_____

_____

_____

Vitamins/Herbs:_____

_____

_____

_____

Today's Diet

Breakfast:_____

_____

_____

_____

Lunch:_____

_____

_____

_____

Dinner:_____

_____

_____

_____

Snacks:_____

_____

Thoughts and Feelings Today

_____
_____
_____
_____
_____
_____
_____
_____
_____
_____
_____
_____
_____
_____
_____
_____
_____
_____
_____
_____
_____
_____
_____
_____
_____
_____
_____

Date:_____Weight:_____BP:_____

Blood sugar level:_____ Hours slept last night:_____

If using a FitBit or other device, number of steps taken today: _____

Exercise: Aerobic_____ Strengthening_____

In general, today I feel: Good_____ Fair_____ Poor_____

Pain level (0–10):_____

Drugs/Medications:_____

_____

_____

_____

Vitamins/Herbs:_____

_____

_____

_____

Today's Diet

Breakfast:_____

_____

_____

_____

Lunch:_____

_____

_____

_____

Dinner:_____

_____

_____

_____

Snacks:_____

_____

_____

Thoughts and Feelings Today

_____

_____

_____

_____

_____

_____

_____

_____

_____

_____

_____

_____

_____

_____

_____

_____

_____

_____

_____

_____

_____

_____

_____

_____

_____

_____

ROSEMARY R. KING APRN, BC

Date:_____Weight:_____BP:_____

Blood sugar level:_____ Hours slept last night:_____

If using a FitBit or other device, number of steps taken today: _____

Exercise: Aerobic_____ Strengthening_____

In general, today I feel: Good_____ Fair_____ Poor_____

Pain level (0–10):_____

Drugs/Medications:_____

_____

_____

_____

Vitamins/Herbs:_____

_____

_____

_____

Today's Diet

Breakfast:_____

_____

_____

_____

_____

Lunch:_____

_____

_____

_____

Dinner:_____

_____

_____

_____

Snacks:_____

_____

Thoughts and Feelings Today

_____

_____

_____

_____

_____

_____

_____

_____

_____

_____

_____

_____

_____

_____

_____

_____

_____

_____

_____

_____

_____

_____

_____

ROSEMARY R. KING APRN, BC

Date:_____Weight:_____BP:_____

Blood sugar level:_____ Hours slept last night:_____

If using a FitBit or other device, number of steps taken today: _____

Exercise: Aerobic_____ Strengthening_____

In general, today I feel: Good_____ Fair_____ Poor_____

Pain level (0–10):_____

Drugs/Medications:_____

_____

_____

_____

Vitamins/Herbs:_____

_____

_____

_____

Today's Diet

Breakfast:_____

_____

_____

_____

Lunch:_____

_____

_____

_____

Dinner:_____

_____

_____

_____

Snacks:_____

_____

_____

Thoughts and Feelings Today

_____

_____

_____

_____

_____

_____

_____

_____

_____

_____

_____

_____

_____

_____

_____

_____

_____

_____

_____

_____

_____

_____

ROSEMARY R. KING APRN, BC

Date:_____ Weight:_____ BP:_____

Blood sugar level:_____ Hours slept last night:_____

If using a FitBit or other device, number of steps taken today: _____

Exercise: Aerobic_____ Strengthening_____

In general, today I feel: Good_____ Fair_____ Poor_____

Pain level (0–10):_____

Drugs/Medications:_____

_____

_____

_____

Vitamins/Herbs:_____

_____

_____

_____

Today's Diet

Breakfast:_____

_____

_____

_____

_____

Lunch:_____

_____

_____

_____

Dinner:_____

_____

_____

_____

Snacks:_____

_____

Thoughts and Feelings Today

_____

_____

_____

_____

_____

_____

_____

_____

_____

_____

_____

_____

_____

_____

_____

_____

_____

_____

_____

_____

_____

_____

_____

_____

_____

_____

ROSEMARY R. KING APRN, BC

Date:_____Weight:_____BP:_____

Blood sugar level:_____ Hours slept last night:_____

If using a FitBit or other device, number of steps taken today: _____

Exercise: Aerobic_____ Strengthening_____

In general, today I feel: Good_____ Fair_____ Poor_____

Pain level (0–10):_____

Drugs/Medications:_____

_____

_____

_____

Vitamins/Herbs:_____

_____

_____

_____

Today's Diet

Breakfast:_____

_____

_____

_____

Lunch:_____

_____

_____

_____

Dinner:_____

_____

_____

_____

Snacks:_____

_____

_____

Thoughts and Feelings Today

_____

_____

_____

_____

_____

_____

_____

_____

_____

_____

_____

_____

_____

_____

_____

_____

_____

_____

_____

_____

_____

_____

_____

ROSEMARY R. KING APRN, BC

Date:_____Weight:_____BP:_____

Blood sugar level:_____ Hours slept last night:_____

If using a FitBit or other device, number of steps taken today: _____

Exercise: Aerobic_____ Strengthening_____

In general, today I feel: Good_____ Fair_____ Poor_____

Pain level (0–10):_____

Drugs/Medications:_____

_____

_____

_____

Vitamins/Herbs:_____

_____

_____

_____

Today's Diet

Breakfast:_____

_____

_____

_____

_____

Lunch:_____

_____

_____

_____

Dinner:_____

_____

_____

_____

Snacks:_____

_____

_____

Thoughts and Feelings Today

_____

_____

_____

_____

_____

_____

_____

_____

_____

_____

_____

_____

_____

_____

_____

_____

_____

_____

_____

_____

_____

_____

_____

ROSEMARY R. KING APRN, BC

Date:_____Weight:_____BP:_____

Blood sugar level:_____ Hours slept last night:_____

If using a FitBit or other device, number of steps taken today: _____

Exercise: Aerobic_____ Strengthening_____

In general, today I feel: Good_____ Fair_____ Poor_____

Pain level (0–10):_____

Drugs/Medications:_____
_____
_____
_____

Vitamins/Herbs:_____
_____
_____
_____

Today's Diet

Breakfast:_____
_____
_____
_____
_____

Lunch:_____
_____
_____
_____

Dinner:_____
_____
_____
_____

Snacks:_____

_____

Thoughts and Feelings Today

_____
_____
_____
_____
_____
_____
_____
_____
_____
_____
_____
_____
_____
_____
_____
_____
_____
_____
_____
_____
_____
_____

ROSEMARY R. KING APRN, BC

Date:_____ Weight:_____ BP:_____

Blood sugar level:_____ Hours slept last night:_____

If using a FitBit or other device, number of steps taken today: _____

Exercise: Aerobic_____ Strengthening_____

In general, today I feel: Good_____ Fair_____ Poor_____

Pain level (0–10):_____

Drugs/Medications:_____

_____

_____

_____

Vitamins/Herbs:_____

_____

_____

_____

Today's Diet

Breakfast:_____

_____

_____

_____

_____

Lunch:_____

_____

_____

_____

Dinner:_____

_____

_____

_____

Snacks:_____

_____

_____

Thoughts and Feelings Today

_____

_____

_____

_____

_____

_____

_____

_____

_____

_____

_____

_____

_____

_____

_____

_____

_____

_____

_____

_____

_____

_____

_____

_____

_____

ROSEMARY R. KING APRN, BC

Date:_____ Weight:_____ BP:_____

Blood sugar level:_____ Hours slept last night:_____

If using a FitBit or other device, number of steps taken today: _____

Exercise: Aerobic_____ Strengthening_____

In general, today I feel: Good_____ Fair_____ Poor_____

Pain level (0–10):_____

Drugs/Medications:_____

_____

_____

_____

Vitamins/Herbs:_____

_____

_____

_____

Today's Diet

Breakfast:_____

_____

_____

_____

Lunch:_____

_____

_____

_____

Dinner:_____

_____

_____

_____

Snacks:_____

_____

_____

Thoughts and Feelings Today

_____

_____

_____

_____

_____

_____

_____

_____

_____

_____

_____

_____

_____

_____

_____

_____

_____

_____

_____

_____

ROSEMARY R. KING APRN, BC

Date:_____ Weight:_____ BP:_____

Blood sugar level:_____ Hours slept last night:_____

If using a FitBit or other device, number of steps taken today: _____

Exercise: Aerobic_____ Strengthening_____

In general, today I feel: Good_____ Fair_____ Poor_____

Pain level (0–10):_____

Drugs/Medications:_____
_____
_____
_____

Vitamins/Herbs:_____
_____
_____
_____

Today's Diet

Breakfast:_____
_____
_____
_____

Lunch:_____
_____
_____
_____

Dinner:_____
_____
_____
_____

Snacks:_____

_____

_____

Thoughts and Feelings Today

_____
_____
_____
_____
_____
_____
_____
_____
_____
_____
_____
_____
_____
_____
_____
_____
_____
_____
_____
_____
_____
_____
_____
_____
_____

ROSEMARY R. KING APRN, BC

APPENDIX A

Questions to Ask Your Doctors

Having been given the *C* word, you will, no doubt, be driven into a whirlwind of tests, x-rays, biopsies, and appointments with many different doctors, each of whom are specialized in a certain aspect of cancer care. You are overwhelmed; your emotions and anxiety are running high; you do not know what is next. Being prepared and learning all you can about your cancer and the possible treatments will only make you feel more confident and put *you* in the driver's seat. I have listed some general questions to consider when meeting with your doctors. More questions will arise, depending upon the answers you get. At least you have something to start with. You may want to copy them and take with you to your appointment.

Suggested questions for the breast-cancer surgeon:

o   What procedure do you recommend (lumpectomy versus mastectomy), and why? Will I need to have reconstructive surgery?

o   Are there other options?

o   What are the benefits and risks of each option?

o   If I choose to do nothing, what will happen?

o   I may want to get a second opinion. Whom would you suggest?

o What preop labs and tests do I need prior to surgery?

o Do I need to stop taking certain medications or stop smoking prior to surgery?

o Is this an outpatient procedure or in-patient? If in-patient, how long would I need to be in the hospital?

o How long is the procedure?

• Will you be taking a sentinel node biopsy at the same time as the procedure? What can I expect from that?

• Do I need to be concerned about lymphedema if you take sentinel nodes? What can be done about that?

o When will I know final results of the pathology? (How big is the cancer; what type is it; are the margins clear; is there evidence of cancer in the sentinel nodes suggesting lymphatic spread; what is the stage; what is the hormone status; what is the HER2 status?) What is my prognosis? What is my chance for survival?

o What type of pain should I expect postoperatively? Nerve pain?

o What are some ordinary complications that I might expect or anticipate? What signs would I need to look for?

o How long is the recovery time? Will there be any restrictions?

o Can I expect permanent effects from the surgery?

o How long will I be off work?

o When will you follow up with me? Is there a way for me to communicate with you (e.g., email or text) if there is a problem?

- Will I need to stop taking birth control pills or hormone-replacement pills after the surgery?

- Will I need any chemotherapy or radiation after my surgery?

Information on your doctor as well as patients' perspective on their quality of care can be found on the internet. Websites that can be accessed include the following:

www.vitals.com
https://www.healthgrades.com
https://doctor.webmd.com

o Is the physician board certified?

o Does the physician specialize in breast cancer surgery?

o What insurance plans does the physician accept?

o On a scale of one to five, what is the average grade given to this physician?

Suggested questions for the oncologist:

o Many of the same questions as above, plus the following.

o What is the hormone status of my tumor? What is my HER2 status?

o What type of chemotherapy do you recommend? Hormonal therapy?

o How long does each treatment last? Will I need to have someone drive me home?

o Can I work, exercise, and have sex during my treatment?

o How long do you think I will need this treatment?

o What are the side effects of this treatment? Common and unusual?

o Will I lose my hair? If so, are there resources for wigs or head coverings?

o Will this affect my ability to have children?

o If I have a history of cancer in my family, will this affect the type of treatment I will need?

o Should I consider clinical trials for my type of cancer?

o What type of diet should I strive for? Supplements?

Suggested questions for the radiation oncologist:

o Many of the same questions as above and the following.

o How many radiation treatments do you recommend? Is this considered curative or palliative?

o What are my five-year and ten-year survival chances, with and without radiation?

o How long does each treatment take? Do I need to bring someone with me?

o What should I wear during treatments?

o What can I do to ease some of the side effects? How will this affect my skin?

o Do I need to stay out of the sun?

o Can I work during treatments? What about restrictions?

o Can I take supplements?

o What kind of diet should I eat?

o If I have radiation now, can I have radiation later if I should have a recurrence?

o Will radiation affect my lungs, heart, and thyroid?

APPENDIX B

Recommended Books

The following list has been highly recommended, either by me or by those in several support groups.

Blaylock, R. *Natural Strategies for Cancer Patients*. New York: Twin Streams, 2003.

Bollinger, T. *The Truth about Cancer*. Carlsbad: Hay House, 2016.

Chan, D. *Breast Cancer: Real Questions, Real Answers*. New York: Marlowe and Co., 2006.

Christofferson, T. *Tripping over the Truth*. White River Junction: Chelsea Green Publishing, 2017.

Desaulneirs, V. *Heal Breast Cancer Naturally*. TCK Publishing, 2014.

Fortson, L. *Embrace, Release, Heal*. Canada, 2011.

Fung, J., and J. Moore. *The Complete Guide to Fasting*. Las Vegas: Victory Belt Publishing, 2016.

Geffen, J. *The Journey through Cancer*. Random House, 2007.

Greger, M. *How Not to Die: Discover the Foods Scientifically Proven to Prevent and Reverse Disease*. New York? Flatiron Books, 2015.

Hrbacek, J. *Cancer Free? Are You Sure?* Texas: Gabar Publishing, 2017.

Kalamian, M. *Keto for Cancer*. White River Junction: Chelsea Green Publishing, 2017.

Kemp, D., and P. Daly. *Ketogenic Kitchen*. White River Junction: Chelsea Green Publishing, 2016.

Kharrazian, D. *Why Do I Still Have Thyroid Symptoms When My Labs Are Normal?* Carlsbad: Elephant Press, 2006.

LeShan, L. *Cancer as a Turning Point*. New York: Penguin Books, 1994.

Link, J., and J. Waisman. *The Breast Cancer Survival Manuel, Sixth ed: A Step-by-Step Guide for Women with Newly Diagnosed Breast Cancer*. New York: St. Martin's Press, 2017.

Lipton, B. *Biology of Belief*. Carlsbad: Hay House, 2005.

Love, S. *Dr. Susan Love's Breast Book*. Da Capo Press, 2015.

Mercola, J. *Fat for Fuel*. Carlsbad: Hay House, 2017.

Murphy, C. *Iscador: Mistletoe in Cancer Therapy*. New York: Lantern Books, 2001.

Nakazawa, D. *The Last Best Cure*. New York: Hudson Street Press, 2013.

Quillin, P. *Beating Cancer with Nutrition*. Carlsbad: Nutrition Times Press, 2005.

Servan-Schreiber, D. *AntiCancer: A New Way of Life*. New York: Penquin Books, 2007.

Seyfried, T. *Cancer as a Metabolic Disease: On the Origin, Management, and Prevention of Cancer*. Hoboken: John Wiley & Sons, 2012.

Shanahan, C. *Deep Nutrition*. New York: Flatiron Books, 2008.

Silver, M. *Breast Cancer Husband: How to Help Your Wife (and Yourself) During Diagnosis, Treatment, and Beyond*. New York: Rodale Books, 2004.

Stengler, M., and P. Anderson. *Outside the Box Cancer Therapies*. Carlsbad: Hay House, 2018.

Stresheim, C. *Defeat Cancer: Fifteen Doctors of Integrative and Naturopathic Medicine Tell You How*. Lake Tahoe: BioMed Publishing, 2011.

Treasure, J. *Cannabis and Cancer*. Ashland: OncoHerb, 2016.

Uspenski, M. *Cancer Hates Tea*. Salem: Page Street Publishing, 2016.

Turner, K. *Radical Remission*. New York: HarperCollins, 2014.

Wiley, T. *Lights Out*. New York: Pocket Books, 2000.

Winters, N., and J. Kelley. *The Metabolic Approach to Cancer*. White River Junction: Chelsea Green Publishing, 2017.

APPENDIX C

Helpful Websites

Alternative and Complementary Treatments

https://breastcancerconqueror.com/about/about-dr-v/

Their statement: "To inspire, support, and connect all women around the globe to live their best life through healing of body, mind, and soul."

http://cannabis-med.org/

Their statement: "The aim of the association is to advance knowledge on cannabis, cannabinoids, the endocannabinoid system, and related topics, especially with regard to their therapeutic potential."

https://www.chrisbeatcancer.com/

Their statement: "Inspires countless people to take control of their health and reverse disease with a radical transformation of diet and lifestyle."

http://www.greenmedinfo.com

Their statement: "Evidence-based natural medicine research."

http://www.healingcancernaturally.com/naturalcancer-curetes

Their statement: "Devoted to the extensive field of alternative non-intrusive healing modalities for cancer that have proven successful for people with this serious challenge."

https://www.leafly.com/

Their statement: "The world's cannabis information resource."

https://www.medicaljane.com/

Their statement: "Medical Jane provides free medical cannabis education and resources to suffering patients who deserve a better quality of life."

http://norml.org/libra … /recent-research-on-medical-marijuana

Their statement: "NORML's mission is to move public opinion sufficiently to legalize the responsible use of marijuana by adults, and to serve as an advocate for consumers to assure they have access to high-quality marijuana that is safe, convenient, and affordable."

https://www.projectcbd.org/

Their statement: "Nonprofit dedicated to promoting and publicizing research into the medical uses of cannabidiol (CBD) and other components of the cannabis plant."

www.RadicalRemission.com

Their statement: "Summarizes her research into the radical remission of cancer—when someone heals from cancer without Western medicine or after Western medicine has failed."

Blogs

http://www.anticancermom.com

Their statement: "A whole-body approach to cancer is the only way a person can truly heal. Permanent changes to your diet, lifestyle, and thinking habits are the only things that will keep cancer from returning."

http://cancercompassalternateroute.com/testimonials/

Their statement: "Blog created to provide information for those who are struggling with cancer and are looking for alternative options."

Financial Assistance

www.cancerfac.org

Their statement: "A coalition of organizations helping cancer patients manage their financial challenges."

General Information

https://bpspubs.onlinelibrary.wiley.com/

Their statement: "The *British Journal of Pharmacology (BJP)* is a broad-based international journal covering all aspects of experimental pharmacology."

www.breastcancer.org

Their statement: "Nonprofit organization dedicated to providing the most reliable, complete, and up-to-date information about breast cancer."

www.cancer.gov

Their statement: "National cancer institute (NCI) is the nation's trusted source for cancer information."

www.cancer.org

Their statement: "On a mission to free the world from cancer. Until we do, we'll be funding and conducting research, sharing expert information, supporting patients, and spreading the word about prevention."

www.cancercare.org/treatment

Their statement: "Provides free professional support services to cope with cancer treatment, as well as reliable cancer information and resources."

www.cancersupportcommunity.org

Their statement: "Is to ensure that all people impacted by cancer are empowered by knowledge, strengthened by action, and sustained by community."

www.Cancertutor.com

Their statement: "Provides informational articles which focus on specific types of cancer and offer a recommended protocol for each."

https://hope4cancer.com/

Their statement: "Our unique cancer treatment centers help patients heal the root causes of cancer while building the foundation for lasting health."

https://www.jci.org/

Their statement: "The journal publishes basic and phase 1/2 clinical research submissions in all biomedical specialties, including autoimmunity, gastroenterology, immunology, metabolism, nephrology, neuroscience, oncology, pulmonology, vascular biology, and many others."

https://ww5.komen.org

Their statement: "Save lives by ensuring that all people receive the care they need and finding breakthroughs to prevent and cure breast cancer."

www.mbcn.org

Their statement: "Educate patients about metastatic breast cancer treatments and how to cope with the disease. Educate the public about the differences between early and advanced stage disease."

https://www.medscape.com

Their statement: "Our mission is to improve patient care with comprehensive clinical information and resources essential to physicians and healthcare professionals."

https://www.ncbi.nlm.nih.gov/pubmed

Their statement: "NCBI's mission is to develop new information technologies to aid in the understanding of fundamental molecular and genetic processes that control health and disease."

www.sharsheret.org

Their statement: "Is a national not-for-profit organization supporting young Jewish women and their families facing breast cancer."

www.sistersnetworkinc.org

Their statement: "Is committed to increasing local and national attention to the devastating impact that breast cancer has in the African American community."

www.supportconnection.org

Their statement: "Not-for-profit organization that provides emotional, social, and educational support to women, their families, and friends affected by breast and ovarian cancer."

https://thetruthaboutcancer.com/

Their statement: "Doctors, researchers, experts, and survivors show you exactly how to prevent and treat cancer."

Lodging

www.joeshouse.org

Their statement: "Joe's House website lists thousands of places to stay across the country near hospitals and treatments centers that offer a discount for traveling patients and their loved ones."

Nutrition

www.cancernutritionconsortium.org

Their statement: "Recognizes the importance of food and nutrition to positive medical outcomes of cancer treatment. Our recipes and recommendations incorporate a wide range of insights."

www.cookforyourlife.org

Their statement: "We teach healthy cooking to people touched by cancer."

https://foodrevolution.org/about-us/

Their statement: "Is committed to healthy, ethical, and sustainable food for all."

www.nutritionfacts.org

Their statement: "Is a strictly non-commercial, science-based public service provided by Dr. Michael Greger, providing free updates on the latest in nutrition research via bite-sized videos. There are more than a thousand videos on nearly every aspect of healthy eating, with new videos and articles uploaded every day."

Transportation

www.aircarealliance.org

Their statement: "More than sixty groups have volunteer pilots who will fly patients for care or provide other flights or aviation services to help those in need or serve our communities."

www.angelwheels.org

Their statement: "Non-profit charity, dedicated to providing non-emergency, long-distance ground transportation to financially disadvantaged, ambulatory patients who are traveling for treatment."

APPENDIX D

Facebook Support Groups

You don't have to go this alone. The following groups are dedicated to breast cancer survivors. I believe all are closed groups, which means that whatever is posted remains solely in that group. This allows for frank discussion as well as personal questions. I have found them to be quite helpful. Groups range in membership to just a few women to thousands. There are groups for DCIS; some are for women with more advanced disease. There are also others are for natural or alternative healing choices. There are also groups for your caregivers, spouse, friends, etc., to help you. I can almost guarantee there is a support group that coincides with your particular situation. Choose the group that can best serve you in support. Don't do this alone.

Listed as of this printing and in no particular order:

- Breast Cancer Sisters Support Group

- Breast Cancer Family, Friends, and Caregiver Support Group

- HER2 Positive Breast Cancer Support and Awareness Group

- Pink Sisters United Breast Cancer Support Group (religion free)

- Breast Cancer Journey Support Group (BCJ Tribe)

- Advanced Breast Cancer Xelada (Capecitabine) Support Group

- Breast Cancer Atheist Support Group

- Lifting Hearts Breast Cancer Support Group

- Young Survivor Sisters Breast Cancer Support Group

- Secondary Breast Cancer Support Group

- Metastatic Breast Cancer Information Sharing and Support Group

- Mary Joan Breast Cancer Support Group

- Breast Cancer Survivors and Supporters Group

- Sister to Sister Breast Support Group

- Metastatic Sisters Breast Cancer Support Group

- ZTA Breast Cancer Support Group

- IVY's Fight for Hope Breast Cancer Support Group

- Marie Montoya's Fight against Breast Cancer Support Group

- Thriving and Surviving Breast Cancer Support Group

- Inflammatory Breast Cancer, Family, and Friends Support Group

- Freed's Breast Cancer Support Group

- The Breast Cancer Support Group "The Raw Truth"

- Boobie Buddies

- Breast Cancer Straight Talk

- Breast Cancer Integrative Healing

- DCIS, Noninvasive Breast Cancer

- Estrogen Positive Breast Cancer

- The Alternative DCIS Breast Cancer Group

- Breast Cancer Support Group

- Closed Metastatic (Stage IV) Breast Cancer Support Group

APPENDIX E

Helpful Apps for Your Phone—All Free

- My Cancer Coach

- Cancers! The Guide to Breast, Lung, Prostate Cancer, Science, Therapy, Diagnosis, Treatment, Update, and Glossary Handbook

- B4BC

- Cancer Therapy Advisor

- Breast Check Now

- Pills on the Go

- iPharmacy

- Breast Cancer: Beyond the Shock

- Care Zone

APPENDIX F

Glossary of Terms You May Encounter in Your Journey

Definitions thanks to https://medical-dictionary.thefreedictionary.com.

A

abscess: An abscess is an enclosed collection of liquefied tissue, known as pus, somewhere in the body. It is the result of the body's defensive reaction to foreign material.

acupuncture:
Acupuncture is one of the main forms of treatment in traditional Chinese medicine. It involves the use of sharp, thin needles that are inserted in the body at very specific points. This process is believed to adjust and alter the body's energy flow into healthier patterns and is used to treat a wide variety of illnesses and health conditions.

adenine: One of the two major purines (the other being guanine) found in both RNA and DNA and also in various free nucleotides.

adenocarcinoma:
A malignant neoplasm of epithelial cells in glandular or gland-like pattern.

adjuvant chemotherapy:
The use of anticancer drugs after or in combination with another form of cancer treatment, as after apparently complete surgical removal of cancer cells. The method is used when there is a significant risk that micrometastasis may still be present.

adrenal gland:
Either of two small, dissimilarly shaped endocrine glands, one located above each kidney, consisting of the cortex, which secretes several steroid hormones, and the medulla, which secretes epinephrine. Also called suprarenal gland.

alkylating agents:
Anticancer agents that work by interfering with the cancer's ability to reproduce itself by damaging the DNA.

alopecia:
Alopecia simply means hair loss (baldness).

amenorrhea:
The absence of menstrual periods is called *amenorrhea*. Primary amenorrhea is the failure to start having a period by the age of sixteen. Secondary amenorrhea is more common and refers to either the temporary or permanent ending of periods in a woman who has menstruated normally in the past. Many women miss a period occasionally. Amenorrhea occurs if a woman misses three or more periods in a row.

amino acid:
Amino acids are small molecules that are used as building blocks for all proteins. Some amino acids are also used in the body for the manufacture of hormones. There are about twenty nutritionally important amino acids, including glutamic acid, glycine, methionine, lysine, tryptophan, serine, and glycine.

androgen:
A steroid hormone, such as testosterone or androsterone, that controls the development and maintenance of masculine characteristics. Also called *androgenic hormone.*

angiogenesis:
The development of new blood vessels from preexisting vessels. Angiogenesis plays a fundamental role in embryonic development, tissue and wound repair, resolution of inflammation, and onset of neoplasia. It is linked to an array of pathological conditions (e.g., cancer, diabetes,retinopathy, rheumatoid arthritis).

anorexia:
Loss of appetite, especially as a result of disease.

ROSEMARY R. KING APRN, BC

antimetabolites:
Drugs that interfere with cancer cell replication.

antitumor antibiotics:
Antitumor antibiotics are drugs used to fight cancer and not infection. Their mechanism of action is to interfere with the DNA to prevent cell division.

apoptosis:
Programmed cell death; deletion of individual cells by fragmentation into membrane-bound particles, which are phagocytized by other cells.

areola:
A small ring of color around a center portion, as about the nipple of the breast or the part of the iris surrounding the pupil of the eye.

aromatase inhibitors:
Any of several drugs that affect the levels of steroids in the blood by inhibiting the enzyme aromatase. Aromatase inhibitors are used especially to lower estrogen levels to control the growth or prevent the recurrence of estrogen-sensitive tumors in post-menopausal women with breast cancer.

arthralgia:
Pain in a joint, especially noninflammatory.

aspiration:
The withdrawal of fluid from a body cavity or a mass (e.g., a cyst) with a needle and a syringe by suction or siphonage.

asymmetrical:
Not straight, uniform, or symmetrical.

atypical hyperplasia:
A nonspecific term for any condition—usually billed as benign—in which cells have abnormal features and are increased in number.

augmentation:
Breast enlargement through mammoplasty.

axilla:
The armpit.

B

benign:
Not cancerous.

bilateral:
Pertaining to both sides.

biomarker:
A physiological substance, such as human chorionic gonadotropin or alpha-fetoprotein, that, when present in abnormal amounts in the serum, may indicate the presence of disease, as that caused by a malignancy.

biopsy:
Removal and examination, usually microscopic, of tissue from the living body, often to determine whether a tumor is malignant or benign; biopsies are also done for diagnosis or disease processes, such as infections.

bone marrow:
The soft, fatty, vascular tissue that fills most bone cavities and is the source of red blood cells and many white blood cells.

bone scan:
Bone scintigraphy nuclear medicine, a method in which a radioactive compound (e.g., 99mTc IDA) is administered and its distribution in the body analyzed by a scintillation camera for increased or decreased uptake in bone, an indicator of infection or malignancy.

brachial plexus:
A network of nerves located in the neck and axilla, composed of the anterior branches of the lower four cervical and first two thoracic spinal nerves and supplying the chest, shoulder, and arm.

breast reconstruction:
Breast reconstruction is a series of surgical procedures performed to recreate a breast. Reconstructions are commonly done after one or both breasts have been removed as a treatment for breast cancer.

C

calcifications:
Small calcium deposits in the breast tissue that can be seen by mammography.

carcinoembryonic antigen (CEA):
An oncofetal glycoprotein antigen originally thought to be specific for adenocarcinoma of the colon, but now known to be found in many other cancers and some nonmalignant conditions. Its primary use is in monitoring the response of patient's cancer treatment.

carcinogen:
A substance that causes cancer. The Environmental Protection Agency of the United States government has three descriptors for classifying human carcinogenic potential: known/likely, cannot be determined, and not likely.

carcinoma:
A malignant new growth made up of epithelial cells tending to infiltrate surrounding tissues and to give rise to metastases. A form of cancer, carcinoma makes up the majority of the cases of malignancies of the breast, uterus, intestinal tract, skin, and tongue.

cellulitis:
Cellulitis is a spreading bacterial infection just below the skin surface. It is most commonly caused by *Streptococcuspyogenes* or *Staphylococcus aureus*.

centigray:
A unit of absorbed radiation dose equal to one hundredth (10^{-2}) of a gray, or one rad.

chemotherapy:
Chemotherapy is treatment of cancer with anticancer drugs.

chemo brain:
Cognitive dysfunction, such as difficulties with memory, attention, or concentration, that results from chemotherapy.

core biopsy:
A large-bore biopsy, most commonly a breast biopsy from a woman with a lesion, which has been deemed suspicious by mammography and subsequently submitted for pathological evaluation.

corpus luteum:
A yellow, progesterone-secreting mass of cells that forms from an ovarian follicle after the release of a mature egg.

cortisol:
A hormone from the adrenal cortex.

cribiform:
A descriptive term referring to a sieve-like histologic pattern in which sheets of epithelial cells are punctuated by gland-like spaces; the cribiform pattern is typical of adenoid cystic carcinoma.

cyst:
An abnormal, closed, epithelium-lined sac in the body that contains a liquid or semisolid substance.

cystosarcoma phylloides:
A spectrum of neoplasms consisting of a mixture of benign epithelium and stroma with variable cellularity and cytologic abnormalities, ranging from benign phyllodes tumors to cystosarcoma phyllodes; most often involves the breast.

cytology:
The study of cells and their origin, structure, function, and pathology.

cytotoxic:
Detrimental or destructive to cells.

D

dense breasts:
Breast tissue that permits little light to pass through on a mammogram. It shows up white on the mammogram, rather than gray on less dense tissue. It is felt that dense breasts may pose a significantly higher risk of breast cancer than less dense breasts.

DNA:
Abbreviation for deoxyribonucleic acid.

doubling time:
The time it takes for the number of cells in a neoplasm to double, with shorter doubling times implying more rapid growth.

ductal carcinoma in situ (DCIS):
A cluster of malignant cells in the mammary ducts that has not spread to surrounding breast tissue. It is the most common noninvasive breast cancer and accounts for 25 percent of all breast cancer diagnoses. If it is left untreated, as many as 50 percent of patients with DCIS will develop invasive cancer. Because these cells grow in the ducts, they develop without forming a palpable mass. In its early stage, this condition can be diagnosed through the use of mammography.

E

edema:
Edema is a condition of abnormally large fluid volume in the circulatory system or in tissues between the body's cells.

EEG (electroencephalogram):
A recording of the electrical changes occurring in the brain, produced by placing electrodes on the scalp and amplifying the electrical potential developed. The EEG shows three main types of wave, called alpha, beta, and delta, which differ in their rates of production. Delta waves are the slowest and are found normally only during sleep.

EKG (electrocardiogram):
A tracing representing the heart's electrical action derived by amplification of the minutely small electrical impulses normally generated by the heart.

embolus:
A clot or other plug, usually part or all of a thrombus, brought by the blood from another vessel and forced into a smaller one, thus obstructing circulation.

estrogen:
Any of several steroid hormones, such as estradiol and estrone, that are produced primarily by the ovaries, stimulate the development and maintenance of female secondary sex characteristics, exert systemic effects, such as the growth and

maturation of long bones, and promote estrus in many female mammals. Estrogens synthesized from plant sources or obtained from horses are used as drugs, primarily to treat estrogen deficiency.

estrogen receptor:
Receptor for estrogens; its presence conveys a better prognosis for breast cancer.

F

fibroadenoma:
Fibroadenomas are benign breast tumors commonly found in young women. *Fibroadenoma* means a tumor composed of glandular and fibrous tissues.

follicle stimulating hormone (FSH):
A hormone that stimulates the growth and maturation of mature eggs in the ovary.

frozen section:
A specimen of tissue that has been quick-frozen, cut by microtome, and stained immediately for rapid diagnosis of possible malignant lesions. A specimen processed in this manner is not satisfactory for detailed study of the cells, but it is valuable because it is quick and gives the surgeon immediate information regarding the malignancy of a piece of tissue.

G

granulocyte stimulating factor (GCSF):
A cytokine secreted by a variety of cell types that stimulates progenitor cells in the bone marrow to produce granulocytes, especially neutrophils.

H

hemangioma:
A benign skin lesion consisting of dense, usually elevated masses of dilated blood vessels.

hemorrhage:
Bleeding.

ROSEMARY R. KING APRN, BC

HER-2/neu:
An oncogene that will lead to more cell growth when expressed.

hormone:
A chemical substance produced in the body that has a specific regulatory effect on the activity of certain cells or organs.

HRT:
Hormone replacement therapy.

human choriogonadotropin (HCG):
Hormone produced by the corpus luteum.

hysterectomy:
Hysterectomy is the surgical removal of the uterus. In a total hysterectomy, the uterus and cervix are removed. In some cases, the fallopian tubes and ovaries are removed along with the uterus (called hysterectomy with bilateral salpingo-oophorectomy). In a subtotal hysterectomy, only the uterus is removed. In a radical hysterectomy, the uterus, cervix, ovaries, oviducts, lymph nodes, and lymph channels are removed. The type of hysterectomy performed depends on the reason for the procedure. In all cases, menstruation stops, and a woman loses the ability to bear children.

I

immunotherapy:
Treatment of disease by inducing, enhancing, or suppressing an immune response.

informed consent:
Consent by a person to undergo a medical procedure, participate in a clinical trial, or be counseled by a professional, such as a social worker or lawyer, after receiving all material information regarding risks, benefits, and alternatives.

in situ:
In its normal place; confined to the site of origin.

intraductal papilloma:
A small, often nonpalpable, benign papilloma arising in a lactiferous duct and frequently causing bleeding from the nipple.

invasive cancer:

Of or relating to a disease or condition that has a tendency to spread, especially into healthy tissue.

L

lactation:

Lactation is the medical term for yielding of milk by the mammary glands, which leads to breastfeeding. Human milk contains the ideal amount of nutrients for the infant and provides important protection from disease through the mother's natural defenses.

lidocaine:

Drug used most commonly for local anesthesia.

lobular carcinoma in situ:

Carcinoma of the breast in which small tumor cells fill preexisting acini within lobules, without invading the surrounding stroma.

lumpectomy:

A lumpectomy is a type of surgery used to treat breast cancer. It is considered "breast-conserving" surgery because in a lumpectomy, only the malignant tumor and a surrounding margin of normal breast tissue are removed. Lymph nodes in the armpit (axilla) also may be removed. This procedure is called *lymph node dissection*.

lymph nodes:

Small, bean-shaped masses of tissue scattered along the lymphatic system that act as filters and immune monitors, removing fluids, bacteria, or cancer cells that travel through the lymph system. Breast cancer cells in the lymph nodes under the arm or in the chest are a sign that the cancer has spread and that it might recur.

lymphedema:

Lymphedema involves blockage of the lymph vessels, with a resulting accumulation of lymphatic fluid in the interstitial tissues of the body. The lymphatic system consists of lymph vessels and lymph nodes throughout the body. The lymph vessels collect lymphatic fluid, which consists of protein, water, fats, and waste from cells. The lymph vessels transport the fluid to the lymph nodes, where waste materials and foreign materials are filtered out from the fluid. The fluid is then returned to the blood. When the vessels are damaged or missing, the lymph fluid cannot move freely throughout the system but accumulates. This accumulation of fluid results in abnormal swelling of the arms(s) or leg(s), and occasionally swelling in other parts of the body.

M

malignant:
Cancerous.

mammogram:
A radiograph of the breast.

mastitis:
Mastitis is an infection of the breast. It usually only occurs in women who are breastfeeding their babies.

metastasis:
A growth of pathogenic microorganisms or of abnormal cells distant from the site primarily involved by the morbid process.

microcalcification:
A tiny, nonpalpable deposit of calcium in breast tissue that is visible on a mammogram. It can be scattered or clustered and can indicate either cancer or benign tissues changes.

micrometastasis:
A stage of metastasis when the secondary tumors are too small to be clinically detected, as in micrometastatic disease.

micropapillary:
Type of DCIS in which the cells filling the duct take the form of finger projections into the center.

mutation:
A change in the nucleotide sequence of the genome of an organism or virus, sometimes resulting in the appearance of a new character or trait not found in the parental type.

myocutaneous flap:
A mass of tissue for grafting, usually including skin, only partially removed from one part of the body so that it retains its own blood supply during transfer to another site.

N

necrosis:
The death of one or more cells in the body, usually with a localized area, as from an interruption of the blood supply to that part.

neuropathy:
Any pathology of the peripheral nerves.

nuclear magnetic resonance (NMR or MRI):
A noninvasive medical diagnostic technique in which the absorption and transmission of high-frequency radio waves are analyzed as they irradiate the hydrogen atoms in water molecules and other tissue components placed in a strong magnetic field. This computerized analysis provides a powerful aid to the diagnosis and treatment planning of many diseases, including cancer.

O

oncogenes:
Genes that contribute to cancerous changes in cells. Oncogenes are mutations of normal cell genes and must work together to cause cancer.

oncology:
The study or science dealing with the physical, chemical, and biologic properties and features of neoplasms, including causation, pathogenesis, and treatment.

oophorectomy:
Removal of the ovaries.

oncoplastic surgery:
Surgery to remove malignant tumors from the body and then sculpt the operated tissue to an esthetically pleasing outcome.

osteoporosis:

The word *osteoporosis* literally means "porous bones." It occurs when bones lose an excessive amount of their protein and mineral content, particularly calcium. Over time, bone mass, and therefore bone strength, is decreased. As a result, bones become fragile and break easily. Even a sneeze or a sudden movement may be enough to break a bone in someone with severe osteoporosis.

P

p53:

A protein that regulates normal cell growth and proliferation and prevents unrestrained division of cells whose DNA has been damaged, as from ultraviolet or ionizing radiation. The absence of function p53, usually resulting from a genetic mutation, increases the risk of developing various cancers.

palliation:

Therapies that reduce symptom severity, but do not cure.

partial breast irradiation:

Radiation to the core of the tumor rather than the entire breast.

pathologist:

A doctor who specializes in the anatomic, structural, and chemical changes that occur with diseases. These doctors function in the laboratory, examining biopsy specimens and regulating studies performed by the hospital laboratories (blood tests, urine tests, etc.). Pathologists also perform autopsies.

pectoralis major:

A large muscle of the upper chest wall that acts on the joint of the shoulder. Thick and fan-shaped, it arises from the clavicle, the sternum, the cartilages of the second to the sixth ribs, and the aponeurosis of the obliquus externus abdominis. It serves to flex, adduct, and medially rotate the arm in the shoulder joint.

phlebitis:

Inflammation of a vein.

pituitary gland:
A small, oval endocrine gland attached to the base of the vertebrate brain and consisting of an anterior and a posterior lobe, the secretions of which control the other endocrine glands and influence growth, metabolism, and maturation.

positron emission tomography (PET) scan:
A computerized diagnostic technique that uses radioactive substances to examine structures of the body. Cancers use more glucose than normal tissue. This type of tool looks at how much glucose the tissue is using.

postmenopausal:
After menopause.

progesterone:
A steroid sex hormone that is the principal progestational agent; it plays a major role in the menstrual cycle.

prognosis:
A forecast of the probable course and outcome of an attack of a disease and the prospects of recovery as indicated by the nature of the disease and the symptoms of the case.

prolactin:
A hormone secreted by the anterior pituitary gland that promotes the growth of breast tissue and stimulates and sustains milk production in postpartum mammals.

prophylactic subcutaneous mastectomy:
Removal of all breast tissue beneath the skin and nipple to decrease any future risk for breast cancer.

prosthesis:
An artificial substitute for a missing part, such as a breast prosthesis.

protocol:
A detailed, written set of instructions to guide the care of a patient or to assist the practitioner in the performance of a procedure.

ptosis:
Drooping.

R

rad:

The unit for the dose absorbed from ionizing radiation, equivalent to 100 ergs per gram of tissue; 100 rad = 1 Gray (Gy).

randomize:

To make random in arrangement, especially in order to control the variables in an experiment.

recurrence:

The return of symptoms after a remission.

remission:

The period during which the symptoms of a disease abate or subside.

RNA:

Ribonucleic acid.

S

selective estrogen receptors modulators (SERMS):

An agent that activates some estrogen receptors but not others, thereby having estrogen-like effects on the target tissues (such as bone) without affecting other tissues that have estrogen receptors.

sentinel node biopsy:

A biopsy of the first lymph node to receive drainage from the tumor, used to determine whether there is a lymphatic metastasis in certain types of cancer. If this node is negative for malignancy, others "upstream" from it are usually also negative.

seroma:

A collection of serum in the body, producing a tumorlike mass.

side effect:

Any reaction to or consequence of a medication or therapy. This can be an effect carried beyond the desired limit, such as hemorrhaging from an anticoagulant, or a reaction unrelated to the primary object of the therapy, such as an anaphylactic reaction to an antibiotic. Usually, although not necessarily, the effect is undesirable; common examples are nausea, dry mouth, dizziness, blood dyscrasia, blurred vision, discolored urine, and tinnitus.

SNP:

A single site in any DNA sequence for which the identity of the nucleotide differs among individuals, often associated with a physiological variation, such as response to a drug, and used as a genetic marker.

staging:

An international standard for the staging of tumors; the systems of the American Joint Committee on Cancer and the International Union against Cancer are now identical. Staging is according to three basic components: primary tumor (T), regional nodes (N), and metastasis (M). Subscripts are used to denote size and degree of involvement; for example, 0 indicates undetectable, and 1, 2, 3, and 4 a progressive increase in size or involvement. Thus, a tumor might be described as $T_1N_2M_0$.

stem cell:

Cells that have the ability to self-replicate and give rise to specialized cells. Stem cells can be found at different stages of fetal development and are present in a wide range of adult tissues. Many of the terms used to distinguish stem cells are based on their origins and the cell types of their progeny.

subareolar abscess:

A subcutaneous abscess of the breast tissue beneath the areola of the nipple.

T

tamoxifen:

A nonsteroidal antiestrogen used in the palliative treatment of advanced breast cancer in premenopausal and postmenopausal women whose tumors are estrogen dependent. Tamoxifen has also been used to reduce the incidence of breast cancer in women with a high risk for developing it and for treating gynecomastia, precocious puberty, and other instances of estrogen excess.

targeted therapy:

A generic term for therapies that have impact on a specific molecular pathway or target.

telomere:
The distal end of a chromosome arm; telomeres undergo dramatic changes during the progression of cancer.

thermography:
A technique wherein an infrared camera photographically portrays the body's surface temperature based on self-emanating infrared radiations; used as a diagnostic aid in the detection of breast tumors and the assessment of rheumatic joints; also used in the study of pain.

titration:
Incremental increase in drug dosage to a level that provides the optimal therapeutic effect.

tomosynthesis:
A digital tomographic imaging technique in which multiple x-rays are used to create a 3-D image, used especially for imaging of the breast.

trauma:
An injury, physical or mental.

tumor:
A new growth of tissue in which cell multiplication is uncontrolled and progressive. Tumors are also called *neoplasms,* which means that they are composed of new and actively growing tissue. Their growth is faster than that of normal tissue, continuing after cessation of the stimuli that evoked the growth and serving no useful physiologic purpose. Tumors are classified in a number of ways, one of the simplest being according to their origin and whether they are malignant or benign.

tumor dormancy:
A tumor that is temporarily inactive.

U

ultrasound:
The use of ultrasonic waves for diagnostic or therapeutic purposes, specifically to image an internal body structure, monitor a developing fetus, or generate localized deep heat to the tissues.

X

xeroradiography:

Radiography using a specially coated charged plate instead of x-ray film, developing with a dry powder rather than liquid chemicals, and transferring the powder image onto paper for a permanent record.

Rosemary King has been a nurse practitioner for more than forty-five years. Her experiences include medical surgical nursing, oncology, emergency room duty, infection control, quality management, and occupational health. She became interested in holistic nursing and integrative health during the past fifteen years and has learned to incorporate those modalities into her own health. She became one in eight women in January 2018 to be diagnosed with breast cancer. She quickly became the patient in the current medical system, with all the twists and turns to maneuver. One of the things that she found solace in was journaling, which allowed her to quietly put her thoughts, emotions, and feelings down on paper. This book was created to help women going through this battle realize that, yes, there is a new day and it is now a new normal but that there is also hope and resolve.

Rosemary lives in Green Valley, Arizona, with her husband and two Airedale terriers, Toby and Nikki. Follow her blogs on her website: www.focusedwellnesssolutions.com.